# PERIPHERAL NERVE BLOCKS

## A Color Atlas

# PERIPHERAL NERVE BLOCKS

## A Color Atlas

Edited by

**Jacques E. Chelly**, M.D., Ph.D.

*Professor and Director of Clinical Research*
*Director of Regional Anesthesia*
*Department of Anesthesiology*
*The University of Texas Medical School at Houston*
*Houston, Texas*

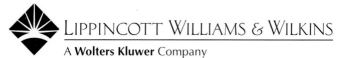

LIPPINCOTT WILLIAMS & WILKINS
A **Wolters Kluwer** Company

Philadelphia • Baltimore • New York • London
Buenos Aires • Hong Kong • Sydney • Tokyo

Acquisitions Editor: Craig Percy
Developmental Editor: Raymond E. Reter
Manufacturing Manager: Timothy Reynolds
Production Manager: Jodi Borgenicht
Production Editor: Karen G. Edmonson
Cover Designer: Patricia Gast
Indexer: Ron Prottsman
Compositor: Lipincott Williams & Wilkins Desktop Division

Printed and bound in China

**Library of Congress Cataloging-in-Publication Data**
Peripheral nerve blocks: a color atlas / edited by Jacques E. Chelly
      p.    cm.
Includes bibliographical references and index.
ISBN 0-7817-1626-8
1. Nerve block Atlases.   I. Chelly, Jacques E.
[DNLM:  1. Nerve Block—methods Atlases.   WO 17 P445 1999]
RD84.P46 1999
617.9'64—dc21
DNLM/DLC
For Library of Congress                                            99-11892
                                                                   CIP

Care has been taken to confirm the accuracy of the information presented and to describe generally accepted practices. However, the authors, editor, and publisher are not responsible for errors or omissions or for any consequences from application of the information in this book and make no warranty, expressed or implied, with respect to the contents of the publication.

The authors, editor, and publisher have exerted every effort to ensure that drug selection and dosage set forth in this text are in accordance with current recommendations and practice at the time of publication. However, in view of ongoing research, changes in government regulations, and the constant flow of information relating to drug therapy and drug reactions, the reader is urged to check the package insert for each drug for any change in indications and dosage and for added warnings and precautions. This is particularly important when the recommended agent is a new or infrequently employed drug.

Some drugs and medical devices presented in this publication have Food and Drug Administration (FDA) clearance for limited use in restricted research settings. It is the responsibility of the health care provider to ascertain the FDA status of each drug or device planned for use in their clinical practice.

*Note:* The following figures have been modified and are being reprinted with permission from Bo WJ, Meschan I, and Krueger WI. *Basic Atlas of Cross-Sectional Anatomy—A Clinical Approach.* Philadelphia: W.B. Saunders Company; 1980.

Fig. 9, p. 24; Fig. 1, p. 30; Fig. 2, p. 40; Fig. 1, p. 46; Fig. 8, p. 49; Fig. 19, p. 54; Fig. 28, p. 59; Fig. 4, p. 75; Fig. 9, p. 79; Fig. 17, p. 85; Fig. 1, p. 90; Fig. 6, p. 96; Fig. 1, p. 102.

The following figure is being reprinted with permission from Gauthier-Lafaye P. *Précis d'anesthesie loco-régionale.* Edition Masson: France; 1985:104.

Fig. 8, p. 24.

# Contents

*v*

**Section III. Continuous Peripheral Blocks**

## Section IV. Pediatric Peripheral Blocks

### A. Overview

### B. Upper Extremity Blocks

### C. Lower Extremity Blocks

### D. Miscellaneous Blocks

# Contributing Authors

**Jean-Marc Bernard, M.D., Ph.D.**  *Department of Anesthesiology,
Polyclinique Jean-Villar, Ave Maryse Bastié, 33523 Bruges-Bordeaux, France*

**Philippe Carré, M.D.**  *Department of Anesthesiology and Intensive Care,
University of Rennes 1, Rennes, France; Staff Anesthesiologist, Department of
Anesthesiology and Intensive Care Service 2, CHRU Pontchaillou, Rue Henri
Le Guilloux, No. 2, 35033 Rennes, France*

**Jacques E. Chelly, M.D., Ph.D., MBA**  *Professor and Director of Clinical
Research, Director of Regional Anesthesia, Department of Anesthesiology, The
University of Texas Medical School at Houston, 6431 Fannin Street, Houston,
Texas 77030-1503*

**Olivier Choquet, M.D.**  *Department of Anesthesiology, Hôpital
de la Conception, 147 boulevard Baille, 13385 Marseille, France*

**Laurent DeLaunay, M.D.**  *Department of Anesthesiology, Clinique Generale,
4 Chemin de la Tour de la Reine, 74000 Annecy, France*

**Sukhijinder Dhother, M.D.**  *Department of Anesthesiology,
The University of Texas Medical School at Houston, 6431 Fannin Street,
Houston, Texas 77030-1503*

**Pierre-Georges Durand, M.D.**  *Consultant, Department of Anesthesiology
and Intensive Care, Hôpital Cardiovasculaire et Pneumologique, Hôpital Louis
Pradel, 28 avenue du Doyen Lépine, BP Lyon-Montchat, 69324 Lyon, France*

**Claude Ecoffey, M.D.**  *Professor, Departments of Anesthesiology and
Intensive Care 2, University of Rennes 1, Rennes, France; Hôpital Pontchaillou, 2
Rue Henri Le Guilloux, 35033 Rennes, France*

**F. Kayser Enneking, M.D.**  *Associate Professor, Departments of
Anesthesiology and Orthopedics, University of Florida, Box 100254 JHMHC,
Gainesville, Florida 32610; Medical Director, Florida Surgical Center,
2001 Southwest 13th Street, Gainesville, Florida 32608*

**Jean Louis Feugeas, M.D.**  *Department of Anesthesiology, Hôpital
de la Conception, 147 boulevard Baille, 13385 Marseille, France*

**Thierry Garnier, M.D.**  *Department of Anesthesiology, Centre Hospitalier
Claude Galien, 20 route de Boussy, 91480 Quincy Sous Senart,
Pontault-Combault, France*

**Louise Gouyet, M.D.**  *Staff Anesthesiologist, Department of Anesthesia,
Hôpital Armand Trousseau, 26 avenue Nettes, 75571 Paris, France*

**Admir Hadžić, M.D., Ph.D.**   *Assistant Professor of Clinical Anesthesiology, Columbia University College of Physicians and Surgeons, New York, New York 10032; Staff Anesthesiologist, Deputy Assistant and Director of Anesthesia, St. Luke's–Roosevelt Hospital Center, 1111 Amsterdam Avenue, New York, New York 10025*

**Carin Hagberg, M.D.**   *Associate Professor, Department of Anesthesiology, The University of Texas Medical School at Houston, 6431 Fannin Street, Houston, Texas 77030; Staff Anesthesiologist, Department of Anesthesiology, Hermann Hospital, 6411 Fannin Street, Houston, Texas 77030*

**Terese T. Horlocker, M.D.**   *Associate Professor, Section Head, Orthopedic Anesthesia, Department of Anesthesiology, Mayo Clinic, 200 First Street, Southwest, Rochester, Minnesota 55905*

**Bernard Komly, M.D.**   *Department of Anesthesiology, Centre Hospitalier Claude Galien, 20 rue de Boussy, 91480 Quincy Sous Senart, Pontault-Combault, France*

**Pascal Leclerc, M.D.**   *Department of Anesthesiology, Centre Hospitalier Claude Galien, 20 rue de Boussy, 91480 Quincy Sous Senart, Pontault-Combault, France*

**Jean-Jacques Lehot, M.D., Ph.D.**   *Professor, Department of Anaesthesiology, UFR RTH Laënnec, Rue Guillaume Paradin, 69008 Lyon, France; Chief, Department of Anesthesia, Hôpital Louis Pradel, 28 avenue du Doyen Lépine, BP Lyon-Montchat, 69394 Lyon, France*

**Gregory A. Liguori, M.D.**   *Assistant Clinical Professor, Department of Anesthesiology, Cornell University Medical College, 1300 York Avenue, New York, New York 10021; Assistant Attending Anesthesiologist, Assistant Scientist, Department of Anesthesiology, Hospital for Special Surgery, 535 East 70th Street, New York, New York 10021*

**Philippe B. Macaire, M.D.**   *Department of Anesthesiology, Polyclinique du Parc Lyon, 84 boulevard des Belges, 69006 Lyon, France*

**Marcos V. Masson, M.D.**   *Associate Professor, Department of Orthopaedic Surgery, The University of Texas Medical School at Houston, 6431 Fannin Street, Houston, Texas 77030; Section Chief, Hand Surgery Section, Park Plaza Hospital, 1313 Hermann Drive, Houston, Texas 77004*

**Maria Matuszczak, M.D.**   *Kliniken der Stadt Koeln, Loeln-Merheim, Ostmerheimer Str. 200, 51109 Koeln, Germany*

**Luc Mercadal, M.D.**   *Department of Anesthesiology Centre Hospitalier Claude Galien, 20 rue de Boussy, 91480 Quincy Sous Senart, Pontault-Combault, France*

**Bertrand Morel, M.D.**   *Department of Anesthesiology, Centre Hospitalier Claude Galien, 20 rue de Boussy, 91480 Quincy Sous Senart, Pontault-Combault, France*

**Gary F. Morris, M.D., FRCPC**   *Clinical Assistant Professor, Department of Anesthesia, University of Saskatchewan, 103 Hospital Drive, Saskatoon, Saskatchewan, Canada S7N 0W8; Department of Anesthesia, Royal University Hospital, 103 Hospital Drive, Saskatchewan, Canada SN7 0W8*

**Vincent Piriou, M.D.**   *Department of Anesthesiology, Hôpital Cardio-vasculaire et Pneumologique, Hôpital Louis Pradel, 28 avenue du Doyen Lépine, 69500 Lyon, France*

**Jeff J. Rockwell, M.D.**   *Director, Acute Pain Management, Austin Anesthesiology Group, LLP, 7706 Blue Lily Drive, Austin, Texas 78759-6406*

**Didier Sciard, M.D.**   *Department of Anesthesiology, Clinique du Sport, 36 boulevard Saint Marcel, 75005 Paris, France*

**Daneshvari Solanki, M.D.**   *Department of Anesthesiology, The University of Texas Medical School at Galveston, 301 University Boulevard, Galveston, Texas 77555-0591*

**Jerry D. Vloka, M.D., Ph.D.**   *Assistant Professor of Clinical Anesthesiology, Columbia University College of Physicians and Surgeons, New York, New York 10032; Attending Anesthesiologist, Director of Regional Anesthesia, St. Luke's–Roosevelt Hospital Center, 1111 Amsterdam Avenue, New York, New York 10025*

# Foreword

The practice of anesthesia requires preparation, attention to detail, and vigilance. It is an accepted tenet of anesthesiologists to administer to the patient the least amount of anesthesia necessary to keep the patient safe and comfortable, and to provide optimal operating conditions. In many instances, peripheral nerve blocks fulfill these requirements. The rapid increase in the ambulatory surgery population has made the present time an ideal one for the growth and development of this form of anesthesia. Although the methodologies for various peripheral nerve blocks have been recognized for many years, the approaches vary, including the use of paresthesias, perivascular techniques, field blocks, and, more recently, the use of a nerve stimulator for the identification of the nerve(s) of interest. For many of us, the problems with employing peripheral nerve blocks are the lack of training and the absence of specific protocols to allow us to accumulate sufficient experience to confidently use a peripheral nerve block as a real option in our anesthetic practice.

*Peripheral Nerve Blocks: A Color Atlas* will help us to overcome these two problems. The objective of this book is to give the reader a simple, practical approach to performing a peripheral nerve block. Therefore, it is purposely limited in its breadth but gives the reader all the necessary information, including the indications for the block, patient positioning, needle orientation, and the appropriate volume and type of local anesthetic solutions to be used. Part I gives the reader a step-by-step approach to a peripheral nerve block and includes information on the proper use of a nerve stimulator and potential local anesthetic solutions and additives. Part II deals with single injection nerve blocks, and Part III considers the important and rapidly developing area of continuous nerve blocks. Part IV is concerned with pediatric peripheral nerve blocks, a subject with which most anesthesiologists are unfamiliar. This book first began as a syllabus for residents at the University of Texas at Houston where it helped to develop a successful regional anesthesia program at that institution. It is now a multiauthored text with contributions from Europe and North America by anesthesiologists who are recognized for their expertise in the practice of regional anesthesia.

This atlas describes and illustrates all necessary anatomical landmarks and specific methodologies of performing each block. The general steps necessary to successfully perform any block are enumerated. Dr. Jacques Chelly emphasizes that the peripheral nerve block, as with every anesthetic, begins with a thorough evaluation of the patient, informed consent, and basic and essential monitoring. In addition, the text describes how to safely initiate and expand one's anesthetic armamentarium to include peripheral nerve blocks. This book will help experienced clinicians expand their practice, and it will help residents and fellows incorporate peripheral nerve blocks into their developing practice of anesthesia.

*Thomas J. J. Blanck, M.D., Ph.D.*
*Director of Anesthesiology*
*Hospital for Special Surgery*
*Professor of Anesthesiology, Physiology and Biophysics*
*Weill College of Medicine of Cornell University*
*New York, New York*

# Preface

In the past few years, we have seen a great increase in the number of the peripheral nerve blocks performed by anesthesiologists. This change is in response to the increased number of patients with ASA physical status III and IV, requiring lower and upper extremity surgery, undergoing same day surgery; to patient preference as an alternative to general anesthesia and/or for preoperative and postoperative pain relief; to surgeons' request and resident education and to economic pressure from managed care. The use of peripheral blocks has been demonstrated to result in earlier discharge of patients.

This book contains a description of the peripheral nerve blocks performed on a daily basis in our operating rooms. Our commitment to the use of peripheral nerve blocks—and the quest for maximizing the success rate as well as minimizing complications—has led us to block our patients before taking them to the operating room. This requires time and organization but allows us to verify that blockade of the appropriate nerves has been achieved, and, if not, it allows us to complete this blockade using a more distal approach. For example, to satisfy the requirement of a surgical procedure below the knee, a sciatic nerve block with an anterior approach at the thigh is performed. If necessary, this may be complemented by a supplemental injection of local anesthetic above the knee after identification of the sciatic nerve. In the case of upper extremity block for a hand surgery requiring the use of a tourniquet, an axillary block or a humeral approach may be used at first and then complemented by a block of the specific nerves at the elbow and at the wrist, if necessary.

To increase the specificity and reliability of our peripheral nerve blocks, we use nerve stimulators specifically designed for this purpose. Thus, a transarterial approach necessitates the performance of axillary blocks. Paresthesia approaches are limited to interscalene supra and infraclavicular, as well as axillary blocks. With a nerve stimulator, it is possible to perform upper and lower extremity blocks. The nerve stimulator is therefore an excellent teaching tool. Also, we maximize the success rate and minimize complications by selecting only certain anatomical approaches for each block.

To maximize success and minimize complications, this book provides the clinician with practical descriptive anatomical landmarks and tips for performing peripheral nerve blocks for surgery and postoperative pain relief. It is our hope that the use of this atlas will improve the clinician's skills and improve patient care while addressing the economic issues of today's healthcare environment.

*Jacques E. Chelly, M.D., Ph.D.*

# SECTION I
# General Concepts

# 1

# Step-by-Step Approach to Peripheral Nerve Blocks

Jacques E. Chelly

Performing blocks in a sedated surgical patient before induction of anesthesia decreases the incidence of complications, and the time spent by the patient in the operating room **(Table 1)**. Regardless of the timing, the following steps are necessary:

1. Obtain a complete and detailed history and physical examination of each patient.

2. Evaluate the indications for peripheral nerve blocks, including preoperative, intraoperative, and postoperative pain control for upper or lower extremities in a cooperative patient and with a willing surgeon **(Fig. 1)**. The contraindications to regional blocks are local (e.g., infection, trauma, preoperative nerve damage), surgical (nerve repair), related to the patient's condition (e.g., uncooperative or unwilling, presence of uncontrolled seizure disorder), and related to the surgeon (unwilling). Coagulopathy, which is often cited as a contraindication to regional anesthesia, should be considered a relative contraindication in the case of peripheral block. Thus, most of the nerves that we block (except for the sciatic nerves) are superficial, and therefore it is always possible to apply compression if necessary.

3. Obtain informed consent by providing a detailed explanation of the respective risks and benefits of general and regional anesthesia. The relative benefit of a peripheral nerve block versus general anesthesia depends on the patient's American Society of Anesthesiologists (ASA) physical status classification. Although it is not documented in the literature, the higher the ASA classification, the more beneficial it is to use peripheral nerve blocks. For the patient to make an informed decision, it is essential for him or her to acknowledge that a peripheral nerve block may be associated with a toxic reaction to the administration of a local anesthetic solution, including seizure, cardiac arrhythmias (related to intravascular injection, increased sensitivity, or excessive concentrations of local anesthetic solutions), and transient or permanent nerve damage (e.g., acute pain during injection, paresthesia, and numbness). The patient also needs to understand that although the risk of physical nerve damage is minimized by the use of a b-beveled needle and a nerve stimulator, this theoretic risk still exists and requires acknowledgment. Finally, the patient needs to understand that the choice of general anesthesia versus peripheral block is not a choice between being asleep and being awake, but rather a risk/benefit decision. Even in the case of peripheral nerve block, the patient can be sedated to the point where he or she is asleep.

4. After consent is obtained, the patient is monitored by blood pressure cuff, electrocardiogram, and pulse oximetry, and the patient's condition is continuously assessed.

5. Choose between single injection and continuous infusion of local anesthetics.

**Table 1.** *Benefits and potential risks of peripheral blocks*

| Benefits | Potential Risks |
|---|---|
| • Consciousness preservation | • Toxicity: cardiac, neurologic, allergic |
| • Hemodynamic stability | • Theoretical increase in permanent or |
| • Post-surgery analgesia | transitional nervous lesions |
| • Early discharge | • Pain and hematoma at punction sites |
| • Better participation | • Discomfort of certain surgeries |
| • Limited sensitive and motor blocks | • Risk of failure |
| | • Incomplete block, if misevaluation |
| | of surgical requirement |

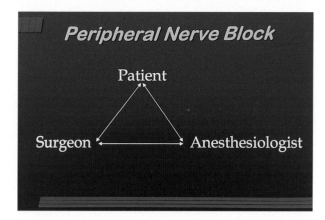

**FIG. 1.**

6. After being properly positioned, the patient is sedated with appropriate doses of midazolam (start with 0.5 mg intravenously [IV] in the elderly and up to 2 mg in a healthy, young patient). The effects of midazolam are potentiated by the addition of fentanyl 50 to 100 µg and droperidol 1.25 to 2.5 µg, according to the patientís response. Midazolam is our drug of choice because of its relatively short half-life, lack of hemodynamic effects, and the availability of a specific antagonist (flumazenil) that can be administered immediately if necessary. To prevent oxygen desaturation, a nasal cannula is often used to deliver $O_2$ 2 to 3 L. It is important to recognize that the level of sedation varies with the type of block. EMLA cream (Astra Pharmaceutical Products, Inc., Westborough, MA) applied 30 to 45 minutes before performing the block provides useful local anesthesia even in adults, allowing a dose reduction of drugs used for sedation.

7. Choose the proper local anesthetic mixture based on the duration of surgery and the need for postoperative pain control.

8. Perform the block. When the appropriate nerve is located, a solution of local anesthetic is injected.

9. Evaluate the quality of the motor block as well as the sensory block with ice and needle pitch after 5 to 15 minutes for the upper extremity and 5 to 30 minutes for the lower extremity. If the block is incomplete, consideration is given to more distal complementary nerve blocks.

10. Before surgery, inform the surgeon of your evaluation of the block and the possible need for local supplementation, and have the surgeon confirm your findings.

11. Instruct the patient in handling postoperative recovery from the block, including pain control relay by oral medication and occurrence of possible side effects and complications.

12. Do a postoperative follow-up by telephone the next day and properly document the absence of complications and the patient's comments. If the patient complains of complications, he or she should return for a complete evaluation.

## SUGGESTED READING

Pavlin DJ, Rapp SE, Polissar NL, Malmgren JA, Koerschgen M, Keyes H. Factors affecting discharge time in adult outpatients. *Anesth Analg* 1998;87:816–826.

# 2

# Nerve Stimulator

Jacques E. Chelly

Originally, peripheral nerve blocks were mostly performed using paresthesia or a blind approach. In some instances, transarterial methods to localize nerves have also been used for axillary and supraclavicular blocks. To produce paresthesia, the needle used for the block needs to be in direct contact with the nerve. Although not proven, this method of nerve localization carries an intrinsic risk of reversible or irreversible nerve damage. The use of a transarterial approach can lead to intra-arterial injection of local anesthetics, development of pseudoaneurysm, and hemorrhage. In contrast, the use of a nerve stimulator does not require the needle to establish direct contact with a nerve or the transfixion of an artery to achieve specific localization of the nerve. In theory, the use of a nerve stimulator decreases the potential for post-traumatic nerve complications, hemorrhage, and local anesthetic toxicity.

In addition, the use of a nerve stimulator increases the specificity of peripheral nerve blockade. The response elicited by the nerve being stimulated results in specific motor response. Hence, nerves can be individually localized and blocked, which increases the reliability of the technique. There has been a growing recognition of the value of the use of the nerve stimulator over paresthesia in performing peripheral nerve blocks. Nerve stimulators are now designed specifically for the purpose of peripheral nerve blockade; equipped with a digital display, they can deliver a wide range of current (0 to 5 mA) at a frequency of 1 or 2 Hz, and can be controlled very precisely in the low current range **(Fig. 1)**. In contrast to general belief, the use of a nerve stimulator *does not* require two people—one operator responsible for localizing the nerve (i.e., holding the insulated, b-beveled needle) and one assistant who controls the use of the nerve stimulator and injects the local anesthetic when the nerve has been appropriately identified. One trained operator is sufficient. The initial approach to localize each nerve is performed with the nerve stimulator delivering a current of 1 to 2 or 5 mA (sciatic nerve blocks). When the expected motor response is elicited, the needle is first reoriented to maximize this response, and then the current intensity is progressively reduced as low as possible ($\leq$0.6 mA). The success of rapid localization of the nerve depends on keeping the needle in a very steady position (which is not always easy, even with experienced operators), and on an ability first to position the needle at the appropriate depth and then finding the best orientation within one plan. In many cases, this is a trial-and-error process, and the intensity of the current has to be increased and decreased as the relationship between the needle and the

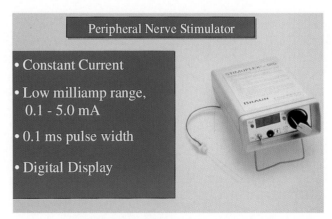

FIG. 1.

nerve changes. It is important to remember to change only one variable at a time (e.g., depth, angle of needle, or voltage intensity). Eventually, the needle is positioned properly and injection of the local anesthetic solution can be considered. At this point, the operator should verify by aspiration that the needle is not placed intravascularly. If aspiration is negative, 1 to 2 ml of the local anesthetic solution is injected, which abolishes the characteristic muscle twitching. This injection is usually painless, but if painful, injection at that site should be discontinued because of intraneural injection and the risk of nerve damage. The time required to perform a block depends not only on the operatorís previous experience, but on the patient characteristics (e.g., morbid obesity, limitation of movements), and on individual variations in nerve position relative to the anatomic landmarks.

The use of b-beveled insulated needles is recommended in most blocks when using the nerve stimulator technique. The negative electrode (black) of the nerve stimulator is connected to the insulated b-beveled needle (N to N: negative to needle) and the positive electrode is connected to the patient and acts as a ground electrode (P to P: positive to patient). There are different sizes of needle, and the size should be chosen according to the location (depth) of the nerve. Only a few companies offer b-beveled needles specifically designed for performing peripheral nerve blockades using a nerve stimulator. For single-injection block and the use of a nerve stimulator, b-beveled insulated Stimuplex needles (B. Braun/McGaw Medical, Bethlehem, PA) are most often used. They are available in lengths of 2.5, 5, 10, and 15 cm (**Fig. 2**). In addition, for continuous infusion, we use the Contiplex Stimuplex catheter (B. Braun/McGaw Medical, Inc.) for the interscalene axillary, supra and infraclavicular and wrist, as well as femoral, lumbar plexus sciatic locations (**Fig. 3**) and the Contiplex insulated Tuohy catheter (B. Braun/McGaw Medical, Inc.) that is available with a Tuohy needle of 10 or 15 cm length (**Fig. 4**). To

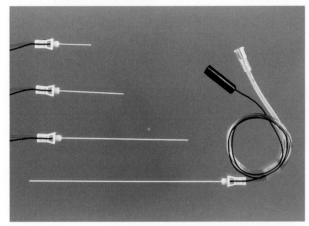

FIG. 2.

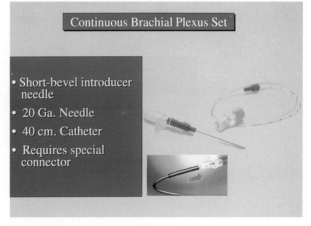

FIG. 3.

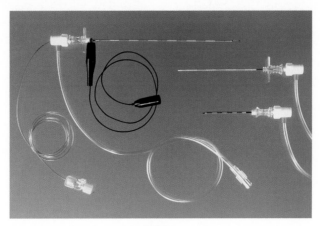

FIG. 4.

maintain optimal control in directing the needle to its appropriate location, it is important to choose the needle size carefully. It is much more difficult to direct the needle if the size chosen is much longer than needed.

There has been considerable debate over the risk/benefit ratio of using a nerve stimulator versus paresthesia and transarterial techniques for upper extremity blocks and even femoral blocks. However, there is a clear consensus favoring the use of the nerve stimulator for high humeral and sciatic nerve blocks. Furthermore, few blocks, such as peribulbar, ankle, and sensory blocks (saphenous block) are performed in the absence of nerve stimulator or paresthesia. Although originally trained in the paresthesia technique, I have found that the nerve stimulator is a more reliable teaching tool and an easier approach to use in patients especially when the concept of paresthesia is difficult to explain, either because of language barriers or intellectual limitations. In addition, the use of a nerve stimulator increases the specificity of peripheral nerve blockade and allows a hyperspecific approach. This produces the stimulated nerve results in specific muscle contractions. Hence, nerves can be individually localized and blocked, which increases the reliability of the technique. A recent literature review demonstrates that nerve stimulator use is gaining momentum in the performance of peripheral nerve blocks.

Although nerve stimulators are primarily used to identify motor nerves, they can also be used to identify sensory nerves. In this case, the duration of the spike needs to be 200 to 400 msec (Stimuplex HNSII, B. Braun/McGaw Medical, Inc.; **Fig. 5**).

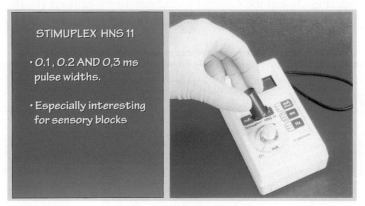

**FIG. 5.**

# 3

# Local Anesthetic
# Solutions

# A. Local Anesthetics

## Jacques E. Chelly

There are a number of local anesthetics available for use with regional anesthesia, including lidocaine, mepivacaine, chloroprocaine, pilocarpine, etidocaine, bupivacaine, tetracaine, and ropivacaine. They each have their advantages and disadvantages as well as different times of onset and durations of action. We have limited our practice to the use of four local anesthetics, lidocaine and mepivacaine (short onset and duration of action) and bupivacaine and ropivacaine (longer onset and duration of action). With the exception of distal blocks, we often add epinephrine to the local anesthetic solutions (premixed solutions containing epinephrine are acidic) to increase the safety margin of each local anesthetic, therefore allowing for a higher recommended maximum dose.

The combination of two local anesthetics such as lidocaine or mepivacaine and bupivacaine or ropivacaine for the blockade of a nerve at multiple sites provides the benefits of both agents: a short onset of action and a duration of action of at least 10 to 12 hours, and often more. Thus, peripheral nerve blocks can be performed without much concern for operating room delays, and adequate postoperative analgesia can be provided without the need for continuous local anesthetic infusions. If longer postoperative analgesia is warranted, a catheter is placed, with the use of a nerve stimulator, before surgery and perfused with a solution of 0.125% bupivacaine or 0.2% ropivacaine at a rate of 10 to 15 ml/hr. Finally, if a short-duration block is required, 1% lidocaine or mepivacaine with epinephrine is indicated.

Lidocaine, mepivacaine, bupivacaine, and ropivacaine can produce central nervous system toxicity (i.e., seizure, loss of consciousness, tinnitus). All local anesthetics (bupivacaine > ropivacaine) can produce cardiac toxicity. Ropivacaine appears to be up to fourfold less toxic than bupivacaine. This lower toxicity is an important consideration for replacing bupivacaine with ropivacaine in our practice. Arrhythmias produced by bupivacaine are often ventricular in nature and associated with fatal outcomes because they are rarely reversible. The toxicity of local anesthetics can be immediate or delayed (within 45 minutes after injection). Consequently, patients need to be monitored carefully for at least 1 hour after injection of local anesthetic solutions. To minimize the toxicity associated with overdosage related to complementary injections made to perfect the block, a waiting period of at least 10 to 20 minutes before a second injection is recommended.

In most cases, we use a combination of 1.5% lidocaine or mepivacaine with epinephrine and 0.5% bupivacaine with epinephrine or 0.75% ropivacaine. We add 1 ml of molar sodium of bicarbonate for every 10 ml of lidocaine to shorten the onset of the block. For upper extremity blocks, this shortens the onset to 5 to 10 minutes. However, it usually takes 10 to 15 minutes for the block to become optimal. For lower extremity blocks, the onset time is longer and varies according to the nerve being blocked. It takes 10 to 15 minutes for a femoral block, and at least 20 to 30 minutes, possibly longer, for a sciatic block.

To minimize complications resulting from intravascular injection of a local anesthetic solution, aspiration should be performed and repeated after each 5 ml of local anesthetic solution injected.

# B. Drugs Added to Local Anesthetics

## Jean-Marc Bernard

**Aims of Coadministration:** 1) to reduce the latency of the block onset, 2) to improve the quality of the block, 3) to prolong the duration of analgesia, and 4) to reduce the doses of local anesthetics.

## EPINEPHRINE

**Site of Action:** Local.

**Mechanisms:** Slowed blood absorption of the local anesthetic agent because epinephrine induces local vasoconstriction.

**Main Effects:** Prolonged duration of the block. Duration may be increased from 30% to 50%, depending on the vasculature at the site of injection. The best effects are obtained with intrapleural anesthesia.

**Other Effects:** Reduction of the inherent toxicity of local anesthetics. Peak plasma concentration may be reduced up to 50%.

**Adverse Effects:** Hemodynamic effects if massive blood absorption or intravascular injection. Tachycardia or arrhythmia indicates an inadvertent intravascular placement of the needle or catheter and necessitates the immediate cessation of local anesthetic injection.

**Dose:** 5 μg/ml (1/200,000).

**Use:** All peripheral blocks, except those in the vicinity of extremities because of terminal arterial blood flow. For example, epinephrine is contraindicated in penis block and usually in arthritic patients or those with scleroderma.

## CLONIDINE

Clonidine is the only $\alpha_2$-agonist used in combination with local anesthetics. It is well documented.

**Site of Action:** Local, but also central after blood absorption from the nerve sheath.

**Mechanisms:** Weak local anesthetic action of the $\alpha_2$-agonist itself, but possibility of synergistic interaction with local anesthetics.

**Main Effects:** Prolonged duration of anesthesia and analgesia that follows neural blockade, depending on the potency of local anesthetics used. Anesthesia may be prolonged by 30% to 50% with mepivacaine supplemented with 150 μg clonidine. Analgesia may be prolonged by 40% to 400% depending on the clonidine dose.

**Other Effects:** Added to lidocaine, clonidine can also reduce the onset time, extend the sensory block, and improve its quality at the time of surgery.

**Adverse Effects:** Sedation is the main and often the sole adverse effect. This must be taken into consideration in a premedicated patient. It is best to avoid premedication or to reduce it in a patient with anxiety over the block. Other effects include decreased blood pressure and slowed heart rate. Rarely, there is an abnormal ventilatory pattern.

**Dose:** The minimum dosage, which results in significant prolongation of anesthesia, is 0.5 μg/kg. Increasing the dose of clonidine results in a greater number of adverse effects. The best compromise is a clonidine dose of 75 μg.

**Use:** All peripheral nerve blocks.

## OPIOIDS

There is cytochemical and behavioral evidence that opioids may have effects on peripheral nerves. Whether such an effect may improve clinical neural blockade and analgesia is debated. Inflammatory phenomena, history of chronic pain, and site of injection might account for controversy. Results are conflicting.

**Site of Action:** Local, but also central.

**Mechanisms:** Hypothetical effect on axonal opioid receptors. Action on spinal cord either by diffusion or by centripetal axonal transport also has been invoked.

**Main Effects:** Analgesia lasting several hours, unrelated to the opioid dose injected.

**Other Effects:** Reduction in the time of block onset using derivatives with high lipid solubility.

**Adverse Effects:** Nausea and vomiting; some cases of pruritus.

**Dose:** For example, 3 to 5 mg morphine could prolong analgesia up to 36 hours. A 50% reduction in the dose of postoperative analgesic may be obtained by adding 0.1 mg/kg morphine to lidocaine.

**Use:** Documented only for brachial plexus blocks.

## SODIUM BICARBONATE

**Site of Action:** Local.

**Mechanisms:** Local anesthetics penetrate nerve cell membranes in their nonionized form and act intracellularly in the ionized form. Because local anesthetics are weak bases, addition of sodium bicarbonate increases their pH to the physiologic range, thus decreasing the ionized/nonionized ratio. This results in both an increased rate of penetration and a greater total mass of local anesthetic in the nerve. An anesthetic effect of bicarbonate itself has also been suggested.

**Main Effects:** There is a 30% to 50% reduction in onset time (i.e., approximately a 4-minute reduction with mepivacaine, 8 minutes with lidocaine, and 14 minutes with bupivacaine). The extent and quality of the block are improved.

**Other Effects:** Prolonged duration of analgesia has also been reported.

**Adverse Effects:** Unknown.

**Dose:** To adjust the pH of local anesthetic solutions to the physiologic range.

**Use:** All peripheral nerve blocks.

## HYALURONIDASE

**Site of Action:** Local.

**Mechanisms:** Enzyme acting on hyaluronic acid, a component of several connective tissues. Hyaluronidase liquefies the interstitial barriers and increases the spread of local anesthetic solutions through tissue planes.

**Effects:** Reduction of onset time (not evaluated).

**Adverse Effects:** Rare cases of allergy.

**Dose:** Not clearly established, from 50 to 150 units.

**Use:** Ophthalmic procedures.

## SUGGESTED READINGS

Bernard JM, Macaire P. Dose-range effects of clonidine added to lidocaine for brachial plexus block. *Anesthesiology* 1997;87:277–284.

Bourke DL, Furman WR. Improved postoperative analgesia with morphine added to axillary block solution. *J Clin Anesth* 1993;5:114–117.

Quinlan JJ, Oleksey K, Murphy FL. Alkalinization of mepivacaine for axillary block. *Anesth Analg* 1992;74:371–374.

Tetzlaff JE, Yoon HJ, Brems J, Javorsky T. Alkalinization of mepivacaine improves the quality of motor block associated with interscalene brachial plexus anesthesia for shoulder surgery. *Reg Anesth* 1995;20:128–132.

Watson D: Hyaluronidase. *Br J Anaesth* 1993;71:422–425.

# SECTION II
# Single-Injection Peripheral Blocks

# 4

# Indications for Upper Extremity Blocks

Laurent DeLaunay and
Jacques E. Chelly

Anesthetic blockade of the upper limb commonly uses a global approach through brachial plexus blockade. Because surgery of the hand does not require complete anesthesia of the upper limb, distal blocks are therefore more appropriate, facilitating rapid discharge of the patient after ambulatory surgery. Techniques of distal blockade of the upper limb nerves are less popular than brachial plexus blocks. Nevertheless, these techniques are extremely helpful and need to be developed. Most of the techniques are described in this atlas. This chapter focuses on providing a basis on which to choose the most appropriate strategy to satisfy the needs of the patient, surgery, and recovery.

## ANATOMIC CONSIDERATIONS

Three factors need to be recognized when considering the role of anatomy in performing a peripheral block of the upper extremity.

### Level Where the Nerves Branch

A radial nerve block performed in the axilla usually results in a sensory block of the posterolateral aspect of the forearm. In contrast, when the radial nerve is blocked at the elbow or lower (below the origin of the posterior cutaneous nerve of the forearm), the motricity of the posterior aspect of the forearm is spared. Similarly, collaterals leave the palmar branch of the median (innervation of the lateral skin of the palm) and ulnar nerves (innervation of the medial skin of the palm) above the wrist flexion crease. Consequently, to achieve a complete sensory block in the median or ulnar territory, the local anesthetic solution needs to be injected at a distance of at least 4 cm from the wrist flexion crease.

### Anastomosis Between Nerves of the Brachial Plexus

Anastomosis may explain, at least in part, individual variations after truncular blocks. To increase the reliability of the block, it is necessary to take this factor into consideration, especially when considering the use of distal specific blocks. **Table 1** lists the most frequent nerve anastomoses.

### Global Innervation

Although in most representations of the upper extremity, innervation is based on superficial distribution, it is important to realize that the muscular and bone innervation is not strictly superimposed **(Fig. 1)**. The only location in which a single nerve

**Table 1.** *Most common anastomoses between the brachial plexus nerves*

|  | Median | Ulnar | Radial |
|---|---|---|---|
| **Musculocutaneous** | Brachial area **Median** | Posterior wrist Upper part of the forearm Hand **Ulnar** | Elbow Palmar, dorsal fingers Collateral nerves Thenar area Posterior wrist |

## BRACHIAL PLEXUS

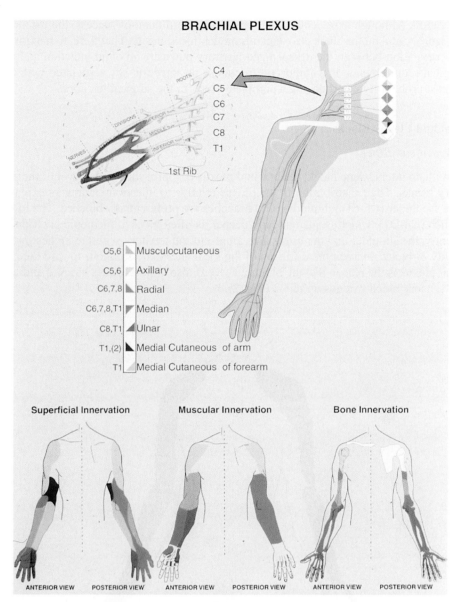

C5,6 Musculocutaneous
C5,6 Axillary
C6,7,8 Radial
C6,7,8,T1 Median
C8,T1 Ulnar
T1,(2) Medial Cutaneous of arm
T1 Medial Cutaneous of forearm

Superficial Innervation     Muscular Innervation     Bone Innervation

ANTERIOR VIEW   POSTERIOR VIEW    ANTERIOR VIEW   POSTERIOR VIEW    ANTERIOR VIEW   POSTERIOR VIEW

**FIG. 1.**

innervates all structures is the lateral edge of the hand and the fifth finger, which are innervated by the ulnar nerve. There are some significant differences between the superficial, muscular, and skeletal innervations. These differences must be taken into account in determining the most appropriate blocks for a specific surgical procedure. Thus, the surgical exploration of a second interdigital wound requires a radial and median block, whereas an ulnar block is also necessary if interosseous muscle exploration is indicated.

## EXTENSION OF UPPER EXTREMITY BLOCKS

Upper extremity nerve conduction can be interrupted at the level of the brachial plexus or the individual nerve. Approaches to the brachial plexus include the interscalene, subclavicular and infraclavicular, and axillary blocks. Others blocks of the upper extremity are truncular (high humeral, elbow, and wrist). Each injection site is associated with a defined probability to achieve a complete block in a given nerve. The orientation of the plexus vis-à-vis the injection site is an important factor to take into consideration. Although experience is an important determinant of success, the extent of the sensory and motor block also depends on the injection site. Therefore, to maximize the correlation between the desensitized territory downstream of an injection and the surgical requirements, it is important to choose an injection site associated with the highest probability of producing a complete block in the surgical territory.

### Brachial Plexus Blocks

#### Interscalene Block

With an interscalene block, the brachial plexus is approached at the level of the primary trunks. Their distribution in the plexus relative to injection landmarks explains why the upper (C5-6) and middle (C7) branches are preferentially blocked. The lower branch (C8-D1), which is anatomically deeper, is often blocked incompletely. Consequently, the shoulder and the upper arm represent the territory with the highest probability of block. In addition, diffusion of the local anesthetic solutions toward the cervical plexus is the reason that the phrenic nerve is also almost always blocked and that the sensory block extends up to C2 **(Fig. 2)**.

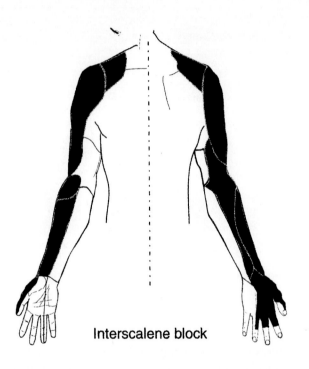

Interscalene block

ANTERIOR VIEW    POSTERIOR VIEW

FIG. 2.

## Subclavicular and Infraclavicular Block

Of all the sites of access to the brachial plexus, supraclavicular injection is the one that allows the greatest diffusion after a single injection, because the brachial plexus cords are very close together at the site of injection. However, subclavicular injection preferentially blocks the axillary, radial, and musculocutaneous nerves because lateral and posterior cords are more superficial. Because the medial cord is more deeply located, the median and, more important, the ulnar nerve have a slower onset and sometimes an incomplete block. Nevertheless, the tangential access to the brachial plexus described in this atlas facilitates the placement of a catheter for continuous infusion **(Fig. 3)**.

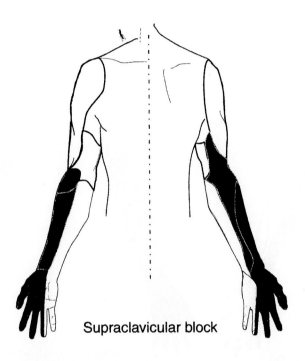

Supraclavicular block

ANTERIOR VIEW     POSTERIOR VIEW

**FIG. 3.**

## Axillary Block

At the level of the axilla, the different nerves of the brachial plexus are individualized. As with the other sites, a single injection does not produce complete upper limb anesthesia because 1) the axillary and musculocutaneous nerves have already left the plexus sheath, and 2) diffusion of the local anesthetic solution can be incomplete. Although there is no anatomically defined separation between the nerves, the presence of fibrous septa limits diffusion of the local anesthetic solution. Therefore, it is difficult to achieve a complete block with a single injection. However, the extent of a block and the success rate can be increased by a multiple-injection technique around the axillary artery (>90%). In this technique, the use of a nerve stimulator greatly facilitates individual nerve localization **(Figs. 4, 5)**.

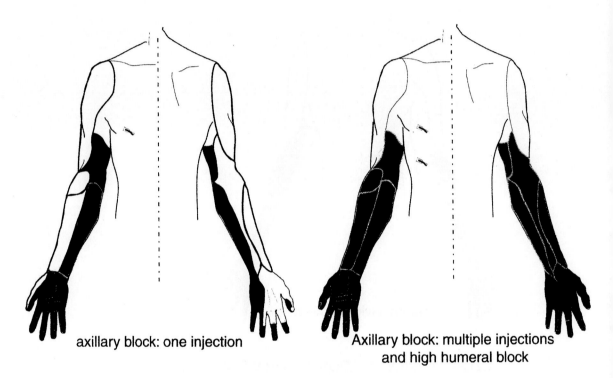

axillary block: one injection

Axillary block: multiple injections and high humeral block

ANTERIOR VIEW    POSTERIOR VIEW

**FIG. 4.**

ANTERIOR VIEW    POSTERIOR VIEW

**FIG. 5.**

## Truncular and Terminal Nerve Blocks

### *Humeral Canal Approach*

At this level, a common vascular–nervous anatomic space exists only between the humeral artery and the median nerve. The other nerves (i.e., radial, ulnar, and musculocutaneous) are completely separated. Therefore, such an approach mandates that each nerve be blocked according to the surgical requirement. In practice, the extent and success rate achieved with this approach are comparable with those in a multiple-injection axillary block.

### *Elbow and Wrist Blocks*

To achieve complete anesthesia below the elbow or the wrist, multiple injections are required. At the elbow, six nerves need to be blocked. Three of these nerves are sus-aponeurotic (musculocutaneous, rear cutaneous radial of the forearm, and middle cutaneous of the forearm) and three are deep (median, ulnar, and radial). At the wrist, or more precisely at the lower third of the forearm, eight nerves provide innervation of the hand and the wrist. Four are sus-aponeurotic (musculocutaneous, cutaneous middle of the forearm, superficial radial, and rear cutaneous radial of the forearm) and four are deep (median, ulnar, front interosseous, and rear interosseous). When a continuous infusion of local anesthetics is required, one or more catheters can be placed in the appropriate sites.

### *Digital Blocks*

The interdigital block corresponds to a local anesthetic infiltration on each side of the P1 base **(Figs. 6 to 8)**. To be effective, it is necessary to block the dorsal and palmar

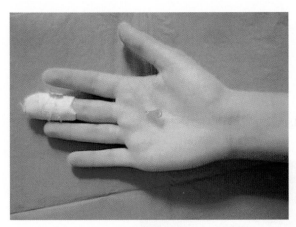

**FIG. 6.**

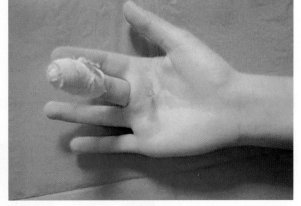

**FIG. 7.**

collateral nerves. The use of epinephrine solutions is contraindicated. In addition, for the second, third, and fourth fingers, the palmer collateral nerves provide innervation to the whole finger on the palmar side and the first two phalanges on the dorsal side **(Fig. 9)**. An injection at or above the flexing tendon sheath facing the metacarpophalangeal joint produces blockade of the collateral palm nerves, thus providing anesthesia of three-fourths of the finger with a single injection. The dorsal surface of the thumb is innervated by the superficial radial nerve, which can be blocked through an injection in the flexor sheath. For the fifth finger, an upper branch of the ulnar nerve innervates the entire dorsal side. In this case, rather than two injections, one in the sheath and one at the level of the ulnar upper branch, it is simpler to make a single injection to block the ulnar nerve at the lower third of the forearm, 5 cm above the wrist.

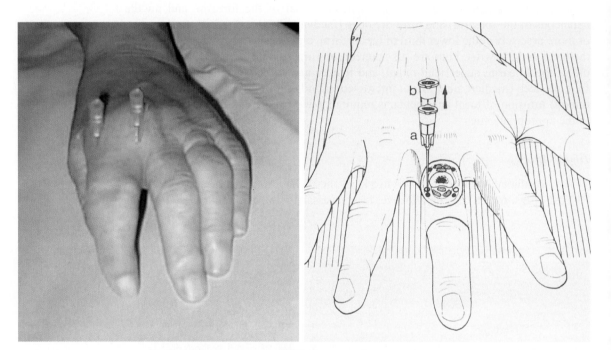

**FIG. 8.**

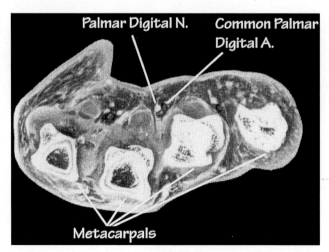

**FIG. 9.**

# SURGICAL INDICATIONS FOR UPPER EXTREMITY BLOCKS

Once the indication for regional anesthesia has been established, it is the location, extent of the surgery, and expected tourniquet duration that guides the choice for the most appropriate technique.

## Shoulder Surgery

The interscalene block is the most appropriate block for shoulder surgery. It can be performed in the absence of general contraindications, including absolute (e.g., allergies to local anesthetics, infections at the injection site, uncontrolled seizure disorder, major coagulation abnormality, noncooperation of patient) and relative (e.g., neurologic abnormalities in the territory affected by surgery), or of specific contraindications (e.g., respiratory insufficiency). If the surgical site also included the subclavicular region, a superficial cervical plexus block is required. Although interscalene block alone is adequate for shoulder arthroscopy and most rotator cuff surgery, some consideration should be given to its combination with general anesthesia. The combination of an interscalene block with general anesthesia is especially attractive when a patient is placed in an uncomfortable position and when surgery is extensive or expected to last for more than 2 hours. In these cases, the block minimizes the use of narcotic analgesics during surgery and the postoperative periods. However, to minimize the risk of complications (intravascular and epidural injections), it is recommended the block be performed before the induction of anesthesia, while the patient is awake and under minimum sedation. If, during the postoperative period, pain control is required for more than 12 hours, consideration should be given to catheter placement. In this case, a high subclavicular access is preferable because with the subclavicular approach there is less risk of secondary displacement of the catheter than with interscalene placement.

## Surgery Above the Elbow

Although some practitioners consider interscalene and subclavicular blocks to be of equal value in patients undergoing surgery below the shoulder and above the elbow, the use of a subclavicular block is most likely to result in a higher success rate. However, the risk of pneumothorax (immediate or delayed) is a contraindication to its use for outpatient surgery. If prolonged postoperative pain control is required, the placement of a catheter is indicated with either a subclavicular or infraclavicular approach.

## Elbow and Forearm Surgery

Axillary blocks using multiple injections or a humeral canal approach yield the best results for surgery at or below the elbow. In contrast, interscalene blocks are not advised given their insufficient extension in the C8-D1 territory. The use of a subclavicular block is possible, but the risk of pneumothorax needs to be balanced against the specific benefit of such an indication. On the other hand, the subclavicular or infraclavicular placement of a catheter for continuous infusion may represent a viable alternative, especially in trauma cases in which upper limb mobilization makes access difficult. Sometimes forearm surgery can also be performed through truncular blocks at the elbow, allowing the selective blockade of nerve territories directly related to the surgery. This requires an appropriate evaluation of the surgical field and determining which nerves need to be blocked according to their distribution. In this highly selective approach, it is important to take into consideration not only the superficial but the muscle and skeletal nerve distribution. However, the requirement for multiple injections may not always be well tolerated by the patient.

Truncular blocks at the elbow are also used to complete the injection of local anesthetic solution at a higher site in the upper limb.

**Hand and Wrist Surgery**

Axillary or humeral canal blocks are the ones most often performed for this indication. A humeral canal block allows the selection of the local anesthetic solution according to the surgical need. For example, bupivacaine can be used to block the

**Table 2.** *Most common upper limb procedures and their proposed peripheral blocks*

| Procedure/Condition | Proposed Peripheral Block | Remarks |
|---|---|---|
| Shoulder surgery | Interscalene block<br>Subclavicular block, especially if a catheter is needed—may be combined with general anesthesia | Interscalene block alone is always possible even for major surgery (total shoulder replacement), but it requires good cooperation between the surgical and anesthesia teams. |
| Epicondylitis | Axillary block—subclavicular block, especially if a catheter is needed | Painful surgery, and a catheter is often required for postoperative pain control. |
| Ulnar neurolysis at the elbow | Axillary block—humeral block | Blocks of the radial and medial cutaneous nerves of the arm are the most important. |
| Forearm arteriovenous fistula | Lateral antebrachial cutaneous nerve block | Injection of 5 ml of local anesthetic solution just deep to the lateral margin of the biceps tendon at the intercondylar line. |
|  | Medial antebrachial cutaneous nerve block | Subcutaneous injection of 5 ml of local anesthetic solution along the elbow crease, beginning at the biceps tendon 4–5 cm laterally. |
| Posterior synovial cyst at the wrist | Axillary block<br>Truncular block at the wrist: radial, ulnar posterior branch, and posterior interosseous nerve | If the duration of surgery is less than 15–20 minutes truncular blocks are an interesting alternative. Do not forget the posterior interosseous nerve, which innerves the articular capsule. |
| Colles fracture | Axillary block | Even for limited surgery, all nerve territories are involved and a complete axillary block is necessary. |
| Carpal tunnel syndrome | Median, ulnar, and cutaneous lateral nerve at the wrist | Musculocutaneous nerve block is useful for endoscopic surgery[a] |
| Dupuytren disease | Axillary block | |
| Trigger finger | Truncular block at the wrist:<br>1. Radial + median blocks<br>2. Median block<br>3 & 4 Median + ulnar blocks<br>5. Ulnar block | Conservation of finger mobility allows for the immediate evaluation of trigger disappearance. |

[a]Median block 6 cm above the wrist, 25-gauge 16-mm needle introduced medial to palmaris longus (6–8 ml of local anesthetic); ulnar block 6 cm above the wrist, 25-gauge 16-mm needle introduced (only 9 mm) below flexor carpi ulnaris tendon (6 ml of local anesthetic); and subcutaneous injection of 2 ml of local anesthetic solution lateral and immediately below the wrist. Wait 10 minutes, evaluate (cold), and if necessary, complement.

nerves directly involved with the surgery, whereas lidocaine is injected in other territories. This may help to limit the duration of the motor block while preserving good postsurgical analgesia. In these conditions, truncular blocks at the elbow and at the lower third of the forearm (at the wrist) may be used to complement incomplete blocks in a specific territory. These blocks have the reputation of being more prone to induce nerve damage, but this has never been established.

The presence of a tourniquet is a more concrete problem. It is usually well tolerated by the patient as long as the duration of inflation is less than 30 minutes. After that, it is necessary to provide additional analgesia via a subcutaneous injection of lidocaine 1% along the medial aspect of the arm to block the intercostobrachial and medial cutaneous nerve of the arm.

Most hand and wrist surgery is ambulatory. In this environment, it is important to maintain good postsurgical analgesia after discharge. This requires a good understanding on the part of the patient about the risks and symptoms of a persistent sensory or motor block (e.g., vascular or nervous compression, wounds, burns). An alternative is to perform a short-duration axillary block using lidocaine completed by a truncular block at the wrist in the territories concerned using bupivacaine. The use of a nerve stimulator is highly recommended. The injection of local anesthetics must be cautiously preceded by the injection of a test dose to prevent intraneural injection. The needle must be slightly withdrawn if there is any doubt.

A number of surgical procedures on the hand can be performed under specific nerve blocks at the wrist (lower third of the forearm). These blocks are better suited for ambulatory surgery. They preserve the mobility of fingers, allow early discharge, and are also better accepted by the patients. However, radial, ulnar, or median blocks at the wrist must be restricted to procedures involving less than 20 to 30 minutes of tourniquet time, and require good cooperation between anesthesiologists and surgeons.

**Table 2** lists the most common procedures in upper limb surgery with proposed peripheral blocks.

## SUGGESTED READINGS

Balas GI. Regional anesthesia for surgery on the shoulder. *Anesth Analg* 1971;55:1036–1041.

Braun C, Henneberger G, Racenberg E. Technique du bloc continu des nerfs au niveau du poignet. *Annales de Chirurgie de la Main* 1992;11:141–145.

Chevaleraud E, Ragot JM, Brunelle E, Dumontier C, Brunelli F. Anesthésie locale digitale par la gaine des fléchisseurs. *Ann Fr Anesth Reanim* 1993;12:237–240.

Chiu TW. Transthecal digital block: flexor tendon sheath used for anesthetic infusion. *J Hand Surg* 1990;15:471–473.

Conn RA, Cofield RH, Byer DE, Linstromberg JW. Interscalene block anesthesia for shoulder surgery. *Clin Orthop* 1987;216:94–98.

Hagenouw RR, Bridenbaugh PO, Egmond J, Stuebing R. Tourniquet pain: a volunteer study. *Anesth Analg* 1986;65:1175–1180.

Hempel V, Van Finck M, Baumgartner E. A longitudinal approach to the brachial plexus for the insertion of cannulas. *Anesth Analg* 1981;60:335–338.

Iskhandar H, Genty A, Rakotondriamahary S, Maurette P. La neurostimulation et bloc axillaire: faut il faire 1,2 ou 3 stimulations pour améliorer le taux de succes. *Ann Fr Anesth Reanim* 1997;16:R147.

Lanz E, Theiss D, Jankovic D. The extend of blockade following various techniques of brachial plexus block. *Anesth Analg* 1983;62:55–58.

Parikh RK, Rymaswzeki LR, Scott NB. Prolonged postoperative analgesia for arthrolysis of the elbow joint. *Br J Anaesth* 1995;74:469–471.

Schroeder LE, Horlocker TT, Schroeder DR. The efficacy of axillary block for surgical procedures about the elbow. *Anesth Analg* 1996;83:747–751.

Tezlaf JE, Yoon HJ, Brems J. Patient acceptance of interscalene block for shoulder surgery. *Reg Anesth* 1993;18:30–33.

Thompson GE, Rorie DK. Functional anatomy of the plexus sheaths. *Anesthesiology* 1983;59:117–122.

Verne TI, Saunders JB de C. Referred pain from skeletal structures. *J Nerv Ment Dis* 1944;99:660–661.

Vester-Andersen T, Christiansen C, Sorensen M, Meisler C. Interscalene brachial plexus block: area of analgesia, complications and blood concentrations of local anesthetics. *Acta Anaesthesiol Scand* 1981;25:81–84.

# 5

# Interscalene Block

Jacques E. Chelly

**Patient Position:** Supine, with head slightly turned away from side where the block is performed.

**Indications:** Shoulder surgery.

**Needle Size:** 22-gauge, 25-mm, b-beveled Stimuplex insulated needle (B. Braun/McGaw Medical, Inc., Bethlehem, PA).

**Volume:** 30 to 40 ml.

**Anatomic Landmarks:** The sternocleidomastoid muscle and the interscalene groove **(Fig. 1).** The sternocleidomastoid muscle is palpated. Posterior to this muscle, the interscalene groove is identified, between the anterior and middle scalene muscles. The needle is introduced at the level of C6 (identified anterior by the location of the cricoid cartilage). Also at this level, the external jugular vein lies on the lateral border of the sternocleidomastoid muscle **(Fig. 2).**

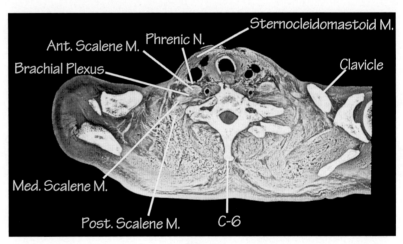

**FIG. 1.**

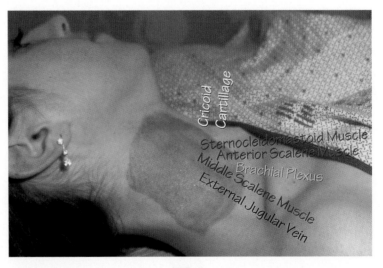

**FIG. 2.**

**Approach and Technique:** At the level of the cricoid cartilage, a needle is inserted into the interscalene groove. The 25-mm b-beveled insulated Stimuplex needle (B. Braun/McGaw Medical, Inc., Bethlehem, PA), connected to a nerve stimulator set up to deliver 1.5 mA, is directed medially as well as caudally and slightly toward the transverse process of C6. Stimulation of the brachial plexus produces movements of the shoulder, biceps, forearm, or the hand involving a plexic stimulation of the musculocutaneous, or radial nerve, or rarely of the ulnar nerve **(Fig. 3).**

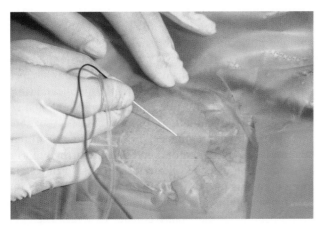

**FIG. 3.**

## TIPS

1. With this approach, block of the brachial plexus is always associated with a block of the phenic nerve and an associated temporary diaphragm paresis. Consequently, this block is contraindicated in patients with respiratory insufficiency.
2. Although the hemidiaphragmatic paresis results in transient respiratory difficulties in most cases with limited consequences in only a few patients, it is psychologically important for the patient to be informed of this possibility before the block is performed.
3. This block is not reliable for hand surgery, and this approach often misses the median and ulnar nerve.
4. Stimulation of the trapezoid muscle indicates that the brachial plexus is anterior.
5. In contrast, stimulation of the diaphragm indicates stimulation of the phrenic nerve and that the brachial plexus is posterior.
6. After injection of the local anesthetic solution, the patient frequently develops Horner's syndrome and a hoarse voice. It is important to inform the patient before performance of the block that this may occur, that it is only transient, and it will disappear as the effects of the block dissipate.
7. Appropriate stimulation of the brachial plexus has to be differentiated from a transmitted contraction of shoulder muscles. Stimulation of the brachial plexus produces movements of the forearm, hand, and fingers characteristic of one of the nerves emerging from the brachial plexus (mostly the radial or musculocutaneous nerve, rarely ulnar).

8. Penetration of the needle into the brachial plexus sheath is sometimes associated with a sensation of loss of resistance ("pop"). However, this does not always occur, and the same impression may be felt when entering other structures of the neck.

9. In the proper position, the injection of local anesthetic solution is easy and is not associated with any increase in the volume of the surrounding skin area. Any increase in volume of the neck during the injection of local anesthetics is suspect and suggests that the solution is not being injected into the brachial plexus sheath.

10. Of all the peripheral nerve blocks performed for anesthesia, this is the block that exposes the patient most to central nervous system (CNS) complications related to direct local diffusion. To identify rapidly sign of CNS toxicity, sedation should be kept at a minimum and the operator should frequently ask the patient to relay any changes in level of consciousness, or a metallic taste in the mouth or ringing in the ears. If any of these symptoms occur, the injection is stopped and 2 to 4 mg midazolam intravenously (IV) or 50 to 200 mg IV thiopental (to prevent the risk of seizures) is injected, and any other necessary symptomatic treatments are started (e.g., oxygen, mask ventilation). In most cases, intubation is not required and symptoms disappear within minutes after the beginning of the treatment. The electrocardiogram is also closely monitored because arrhythmias may occur.

11. If anesthesia needs to be extended posteriorly, block of the suprascapular nerve can be performed for this purpose, and the patient needs to sit up. The midpoint of the spine of the scapula is identified and a 50-mm b-beveled insulated needle is introduced perpendicular until bony contact is made. The needle is carefully moved in search of the suprascapular notch. The proximity of the nerve produces muscle contractions, at which point 7 ml of 0.5% bupivacaine is injected.

12. Do not introduce the needle in a position parallel to C6 **(Fig. 4)**.

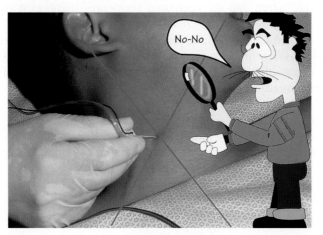

**FIG. 4.**

## SUGGESTED READINGS

Conn RA, Cofield RH, Byer DE, Linstromberg JW. Interscalene block anesthesia for shoulder surgery. *Clin Orthop* 1997;216:94–98.

Heffington CA, Thompson RC Jr. The use of interscalene block anesthesia for manipulative reduction of fractures and dislocations of the upper extremities. *J Bone Joint Surg* 1973;55:83–86.

Urmey WF, Talts KH, Sharrock NE. One hundred percent incidence of hemidiaphragmatic paresis associated with interscalene brachial plexus anesthesia as diagnosed by ultrasonography. *Anesth Analg* 1991;72:498–503.

Urmey WF, Grossi P, Sharrock NE, Stanton J, Gloeggler PJ. Digital pressure during interscalene block is clinically ineffective in preventing anesthetic spread to the cervical plexus. *Anesth Analg* 1996;83:366–370.

Winnie AP. Interscalene brachial plexus block. *Anesth Analg* 1970;49:455–466.

# 6

# Supraclavicular Block

Maria Matuszczak

**Patient Position:** Thirty percent supine upright position, head slightly turned in direction opposite to the side to be blocked, shoulder pushed caudally with the arm straightened beside the body, with the anesthesiologist beside the patient near the upper arm to be blocked.

**Indications:** Surgery below the shoulder.

**Needle Size:** 22-gauge, 50-mm b-beveled Stimuplex insulated needle (B. Braun/McGaw Medical, Inc., Bethlehem, PA).

**Anatomic Landmarks:** There are two anatomic landmarks for the supraclavicular block:

- Subclavian artery in the supraclavicular fossa, at the middle of the clavicle (where the subclavian artery and the brachial plexus leave the interscalene groove and passes over the first rib; **Fig. 1**).
- Clavicular insertion of the lateral border of the sternocleidomastoid muscle.

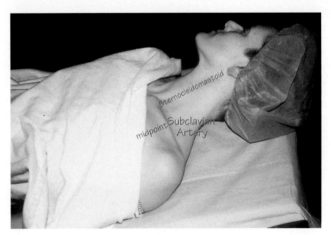

**FIG. 1.**

**Approach and Technique:** With one index finger on the subclavian artery, the 50-mm b-beveled insulated Stimuplex needle (B. Braun/McGaw Medical, Inc., Bethlehem, PA), connected to a nerve stimulator set up to deliver 2.5 mA, is introduced immediately posterior and lateral to the subclavian artery. The needle is advanced parallel to the patient's neck, and the brachial plexus is identified with the use of a nerve stimulator at a current of 0.5 to 0.6 mA at 2.5 cm depth after the appropriate positioning of the needle (e.g., nerve-mediated muscle movement below the elbow: radial, median, or ulnar nerve). With negative aspiration for blood, a solution of 20 to 40 ml of local anesthetic is injected **(Fig. 2)**.

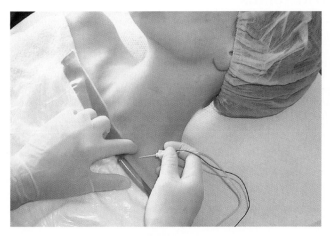

**FIG. 2.**

## TIPS

1. The 30% upright position allows the shoulder to fall and therefore allows a better exposure of the anatomic site.
2. This block is contraindicated in a patient with severe pulmonary disease, or with status postcontralateral pneumonectomy, because of the risk of pneumothorax (with this approach, the risk is estimated to be <0.1%).
3. The first rib is normally reached at a depth of 3 to 4 cm. If the brachial plexus is not identified before contact with the rib, it can be found by walking the needle laterally on the first rib.
4. Remember that immediately medial to the first rib is the cupula of the lung.
5. In a very obese patient, the distance from the skin to the rib might be 7.5 cm or more.
6. If it is impossible to palpate the artery, Doppler ultrasonography can be used, or the needle should be inserted at least 1.5 cm lateral from the border of the sternocleidomastoid muscle (anatomic landmark can be found by asking the patient to push his or her forehead against the anesthesiologist's hand) and at 1.5 cm posterior from the clavicle.
7. In most cases, the clavicular insertion of the lateral border of the sternocleidomastoid muscle is close to the middle of the clavicle; for some patients, it is the point between the medial one-third and lateral two-thirds of the clavicle.

8. Injection of local anesthetic is more likely to result in block of all nerves (median, radial, ulnar, and musculocutaneous) if the brachial plexus is identified through stimulation of the median trunk.

9. If a patient starts to cough during puncture, this most likely indicates the pleura has been irritated and perhaps violated; lateral repositioning of the needle is necessary.

10. If the patient complains about shoulder pain or difficulty breathing, close monitoring and a chest radiograph are necessary to eliminate the presence of a pneumothorax.

### SUGGESTED READINGS

Brown DL, Cahill DR, Bridenbaugh LD. Supraclavicular nerve block: anatomic analysis of a method to prevent pneumothorax. *Anesth Analg* 1993;76:530–534.

Korbon GA, Carron H, Lander CJ. First rib palpation: a safer, easier technique for supraclavicular brachial plexus block. *Anesth Analg* 1989;68:682–685.

Moorthy SS, Schmidt SI, Dierdorf SF, Rosenfeld SH, Anagnostou JM. A supraclavicular lateral paravascular approach for brachial plexus regional anesthesia. *Anesth Analg* 1991;72:241–244.

Winnie AP, Collins VJ. The subclavian perivascular technique of brachial plexus anesthesia. *Anesthesiology* 1964;25:353–363.

# 7

# Axillary Block

Jacques E. Chelly

**Patient Position:** Arm abducted at the shoulder with or without the arm flexed at 90-degree angle.

**Indications:** Surgical procedures at the elbow and below (hand and forearm).

**Needle Size:** 22-gauge, 50-mm insulated b-beveled Stimuplex needle (B. Braun/McGaw Medical, Inc., Bethlehem, PA).

**Volume:** 30 to 40 ml.

**Anatomic Landmarks:** Axillary artery into the middle to lower portion of the axilla **(Figs. 1, 2)**.

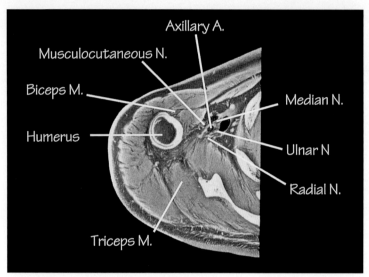

**FIG. 1.**

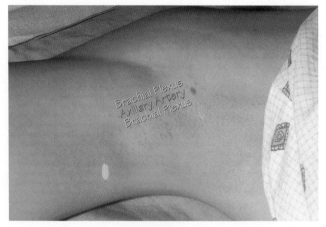

**FIG. 2.**

**Approach and Technique:** At the midaxillary region, palpate for the axillary artery pulse. Once identified, the course of the artery is followed to the lower axilla. At the middle to lower position of the axillary hair patch, insert above the artery the 50-mm insulated Stimuplex needle (B. Braun/McGaw Medical, Inc., Bethlehem, PA), connected to a nerve stimulator set to deliver 1.5 mA. The needle is directed at a 45-degree angle in search of the musculocutaneous nerve using a nerve stimulator **(Figs. 3 to 5).** Half of the anesthetic solution is injected after identification of the nerve.

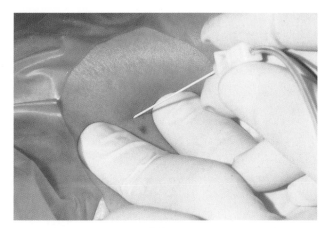

**FIG. 3.**

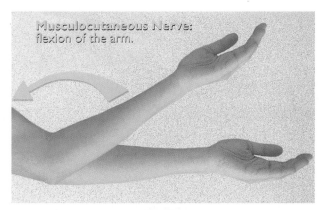

**FIG. 4.**

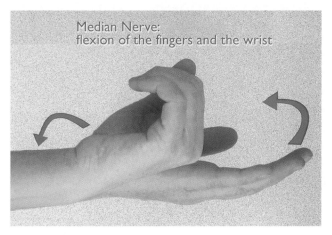

**FIG. 5.**

After injection, the needle is removed and inserted below the artery in search of the radial or ulnar nerve. When the nerve is properly identified, the rest of the local anesthetic solution is injected **(Figs. 6 to 8)**.

After 10 to 15 minutes, the quality of the block is evaluated. If it is not complete, an individual nerve block may be performed with a high-humeral, elbow, or wrist approach, depending on surgical requirements.

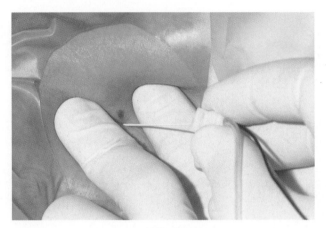

**FIG. 6.**

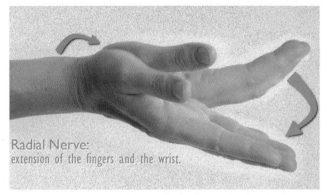

**FIG. 7.**

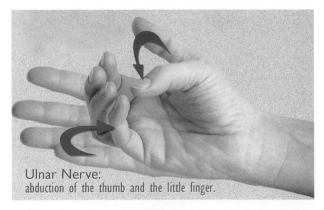

**FIG. 8.**

## TIPS

1. The musculocutaneous nerve may be blocked along with the other nerves with a single injection if the injection of local anesthetic is made high enough in the axilla. However, such an approach does not yield as high a success rate as the previously described approach.
2. The relative position of the different nerves around the axillary artery is variable. In the most frequent distribution, the median nerve is above, the radial nerve is behind, and the ulnar is below the axillary artery.
3. After the first injection, the search for the second nerve has to be done quickly before the local anesthetic solution has had time to diffuse.
4. Digital pressure applied immediately distal to the needle increases the central spread of the local anesthetic solution.
5. To increase success rate, each nerve can be identified using a nerve stimulator, and 8 ml of local anesthetic solution injected to block each nerve.
6. The musculocutaneous nerve is the most distal nerve and does not run with the median, ulnar, and radial nreves.

## SUGGESTED READINGS

Bouaziz H, Narchi P, Mercier FJ, Khoury, Poirier T, Benhamou D. The use of a selective axillary nerve block for outpatient hand surgery. *Anesth Analg* 1998;86:746–748.

DeJong CRH. Axillary block of the brachial plexus. *Anesthesiology* 1961;22:215–225.

Goldberg ME, Gregg C, Larijani GE, Norris MC, Marr AT, Seltzer JL. A comparison of three methods of axillary approach to brachial plexus blockade for upper extremity surgery. *Anesthesiology* 1987;66:814–816.

Lavoie J, Martin R, Terault JP, Core D, Colas MJ. Axillary plexus block using a peripheral nerve stimulator: single or multiple injections. *Can J Anaesth* 1992;39:583–586.

Partridge BL, Katz J, Benirschke K. Functional anatomy of the brachial plexus sheath: implications for anesthesia. *Anesthesiology* 1987;66:743–747.

Schroeder LE, Horlocker TE, Schroeder DR. The efficacy of axillary block for surgical procedures about the elbow. *Anesth Analg* 1996;83:747–751.

Thompson GE, Rorie DK. Functional anatomy of the brachial plexus sheaths. *Anesthesiology* 1983;59:117–122.

Winnie AP, Radonjic R, Akkineni SR, Durrani Z. Factors influencing distribution of local anesthetic injected into the brachial plexus sheath. *Anesth Analg* 1979;58:225–234.

# 8

# Truncular and Terminal Nerve Blocks

# A. High Humeral Approach

## Jacques E. Chelly

**Patient Position:** The patient's arm should be abducted at the shoulder with or without the arm flexed at a 90-degree angle.

**Indications:** Surgery at or below the elbow.

**Needle Size:** 21-gauge, 100-mm b-beveled Stimuplex insulated needle (B. Braun/McGaw Medical, Inc., Bethlehem, PA).

**Volume:** 7 to 8 ml per nerve.

**Anatomic Landmarks:** Upper one-third of forearm and the brachial artery **(Fig. 1)**. (The closer to the elbow, the more nerves are separated; **Fig. 2.**)

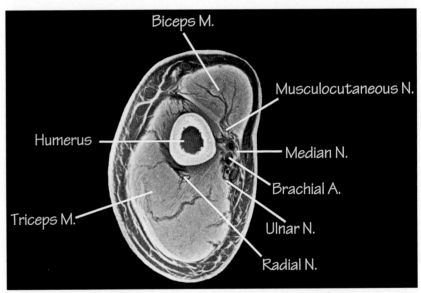

**FIG. 1.**

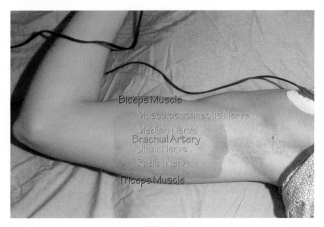

FIG. 2.

**Approach and Technique:** With the arm in lateral extension: (a) the median nerve is palpated superficially above the brachial artery **(Fig. 3)**; (b) the musculocutaneous nerve is located above the median nerve and deeper into the coracobrachialis muscle; (c) the ulnar nerve is reached below the median nerve; and (d) the radial nerve is found in same direction as the ulnar nerve but deeper toward the humerus. This approach allows the nerves to be blocked individually with only single needle stick through the skin. With the arm in lateral extension, the median nerve is palpated above the humeral artery. A 50-mm insulated Stimuplex needle (B. Braun/McGaw Medical, Inc., Bethlehem, PA), connected to a nerve stimulator set to deliver 15 mA, is introduced perpendicularly to the skin. Stimulation of the median nerve results in flexion of the fingers

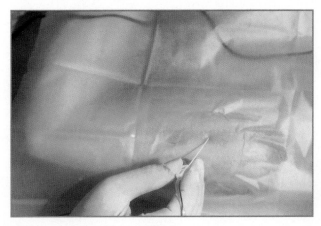

FIG. 3.

and pronation of the wrist **(Fig. 4)**. When the needle is properly positioned, 5 to 6 ml of local anesthetic is injected. To localize the ulnar nerve, the insulated needle is angled 45° downward and directed 1.5 to 2 cm deeper. Stimulation of the ulnar nerve produces prehension by the little finger and the thumb associated with supination of the wrist (as opposed to thumb adduction due to stimulation of the median nerve; **Fig. 5**). Another 7 to 8 ml of local anesthetic is then injected. Then the insulated needle is angled 30° and further directed downward until contact with bone is made. At this point, if stimulation of the radial nerve is not elicited (extension of the fingers, especially the thumb and wrist), the patient's hand should be rotated 30° out to expose better the radial nerve **(Fig. 6)**. At low stimulation current, only extension of the thumb may occur. If so, the arm needs to be rotated laterally to expose the radial nerve. After injecting 7 to 8 ml of local anesthetic, reposition the needle toward the biceps at an angle of 10° upward until flexion of the forearm occurs, indicating stimulation of the musculocutaneous nerve **(Fig. 7)**. When the needle is positioned properly, inject 7 to 8 ml of local anesthetic. Before removing the needle, inject 5 ml of local anesthetic upward and downward in the subcutaneous tissue to anesthetize the cutaneous branch of the brachial nerve. This helps to alleviate tourniquet pain. Installation of the block occurs within 5 to 10 minutes and is tested with cold, puncture, and evaluation of motor block intensity.

The musculocutaneous nerve is tested on the exterior part of the forearm. The radial nerve is tested on the posterior part of the hand. The ulnar nerve is tested on the medial part of the hand and little finger. The median nerve is tested on the palm of the hand. If the intensity of the block is not adequate in one or more territories, it may be completed at the elbow or wrist.

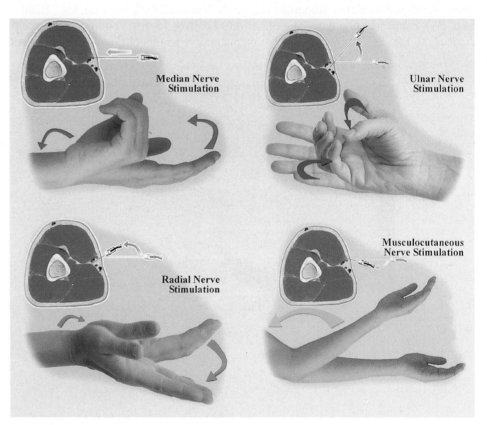

Median Nerve Stimulation

Ulnar Nerve Stimulation

Radial Nerve Stimulation

Musculocutaneous Nerve Stimulation

**FIGS. 4 to 7.**

## SUGGESTED READINGS

Bouaziz H, Narchi P, Mercier FJ, et al. Comparison between conventional axillary block and a new approach at the midhumeral level. *Anesth Analg* 1997;84:1058–1062.

Dupré LJ. Bloc du plexus brachial au canal huméral. *Cah Anesthesiol* 1994;42:767–769.

# B. Blocks at the Elbow

## Jacques E. Chelly

**Patient Position:** The patient is placed in the supine position with the arm supinated and abducted 90 degrees at the shoulder. If blockade of the ulnar nerve is required, the forearm should also be flexed on the arm approximately 30 degrees to identify the ulnar groove. Care should be taken to identify and label the location of the medial and lateral epicondyles of the humerus.

**Indications:** Forearm and hand surgery.

**Needle Size:** 24-gauge, 25-mm b-beveled Stimuplex insulated needle (B. Braun/ McGaw Medical, Inc., Bethlehem, PA).

**Volume:** 4 to 6 ml per nerve.

## ANATOMIC LANDMARKS (FIG. 8)

### Ulnar Nerve

The ulnar nerve is located between the medial epicondyle of the humerus and the olecranon process in the ulnar groove **(Fig. 9)**.

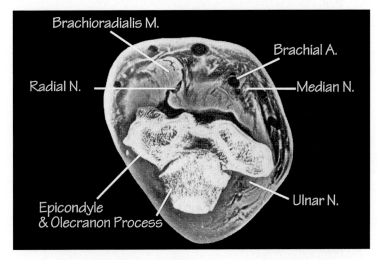

**FIG. 8.**

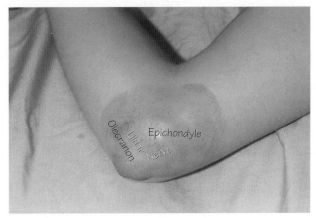

**FIG. 9.**

### Median Nerve

The median nerve is just medial to the brachial artery **(Fig. 10)**.

### Radial Nerve

The radial nerve is just lateral to the biceps tendon at the intercondylar fold **(Fig. 11)**.

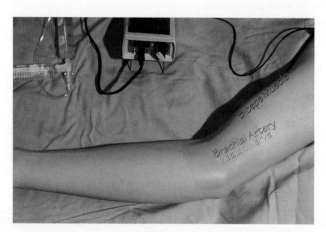

**FIG. 10.**

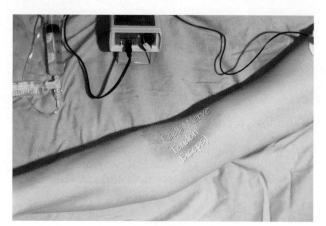

**FIG. 11.**

# APPROACH AND TECHNIQUE

## Ulnar Block (Figs. 12 to 14)

After the ulnar groove has been identified, a 25-mm b-beveled insulated Stimuplex needle (B. Braun/McGaw Medical, Inc., Bethlehem, PA), connected to a nerve stimulator set to deliver 1.5 mA, is placed approximately 3 cm proximal to the line between the olecranon and medial epicondyle. The needle is directed along the longitudinal axis of the humerus. Injection of the local anesthetic solution in the ulnar groove at the elbow can cause compression of the nerve and postoperative paresthesia.

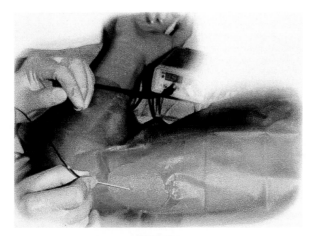

**FIG. 12.**

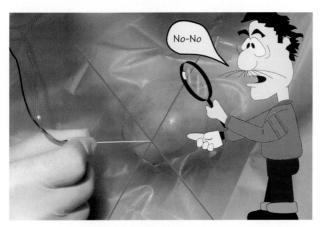

**FIG. 13.**

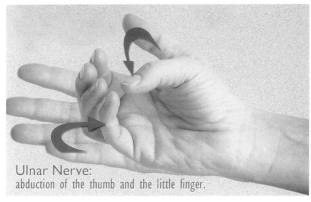

**FIG. 14.**

### Median Nerve

The needle is inserted medial to the brachial artery at a depth of 1.5 to 2 cm. Before injection of the local anesthetic solution, the nerve is properly localized with the nerve stimulator **(Figs. 15, 16)**.

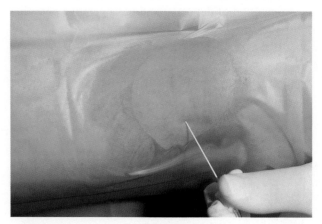

**FIG. 15.**

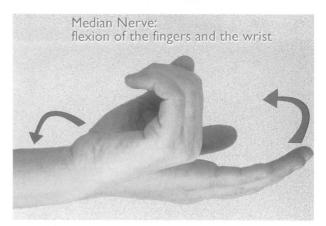

**FIG. 16.**

**Radial Nerve**

After identifying the biceps tendon, the insulated needle is inserted to a depth of approximately 1.5 to 2 cm, just lateral to the biceps tendon in the intercondylar fold **(Figs. 17, 18)**.

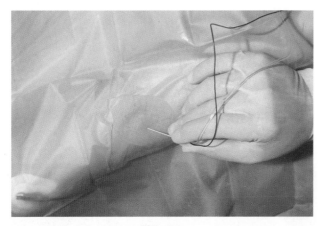

**FIG. 17.**

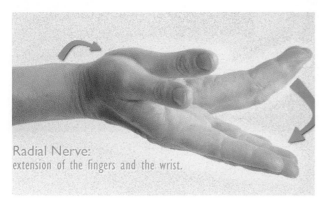

**FIG. 18.**

**SUGGESTED READINGS**

Bouaziz H, Narch P, Mercier FJ, et al. Comparison between conventional axillary block and a new approach at the midhumeral level. *Anesth Analg* 1997;84:1058–1062.

Dupré LJ. Bloc du plexus brachial au canal huméral. *Cah Anesthesiol* 1994;42:767–769.

# C. Blocks at the Wrist

## Jacques E. Chelly

**Patient Position:** With the patient in supine position, the arm is placed with the palm facing upward.

**Indications:** Hand surgery.

**Needle Size:** 24-gauge, 25-mm b-beveled Stimuplex insulated needle (B. Braun/McGaw Medical, Inc., Bethlehem, PA).

**Volume:** 3 to 4 ml per nerve.

### ANATOMIC LANDMARKS (FIG. 19)

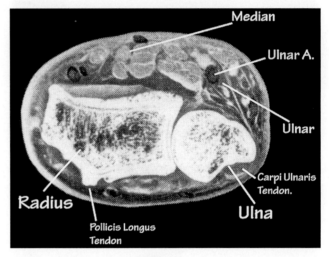

**FIG. 19.**

### Ulnar Nerve

The ulnar nerve is medial to the ulnar artery and below the flexor carpi ulnaris tendon **(Fig. 20)**.

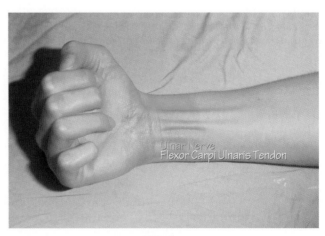

**FIG. 20.**

## Median Nerve

The median nerve is located lateral to the palmaris longus tendon and medial to flexor carpi radialis tendon **(Fig. 21)**.

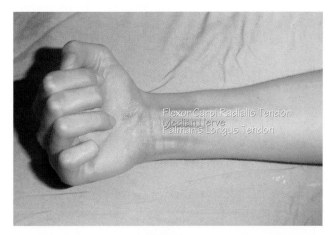

**FIG. 21.**

## Radial Nerve

The radial nerve is just above the radial artery in the anatomic snuffbox **(Fig. 22)**.

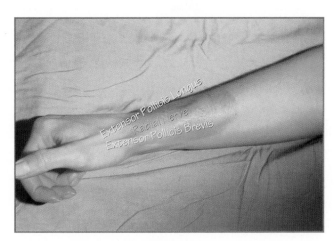

**FIG. 22.**

## APPROACH AND TECHNIQUE

### Ulnar Nerve

After palpating the ulnar artery, introduce the 25-mm b-beveled insulated Stimuplex needle (B. Braun/McGaw Medical, Inc., Bethlehem, PA), connected to a nerve stimulator set to deliver 1.5 mA, medial to the pulse of the artery at 3 cm from the level of the wrist crease. If the arterial pulse cannot be felt, introduce the needle lateral to the flexor carpi ulnaris tendon at the level of the wrist crease, with the needle angled approximately 30 degrees. The ulnar nerve can also be approached laterally **(Figs. 23, 24)**.

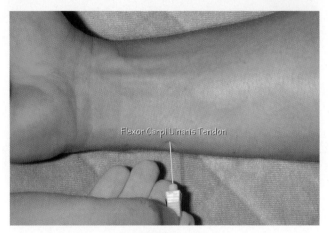

**FIG. 23.**

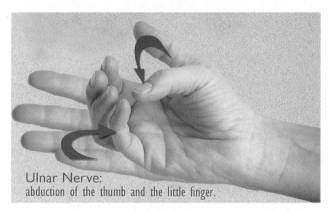

**FIG. 24.**

**Median Nerve**

Introduce the needle deep to the palmaris longus tendon **(Figs. 25, 26)**.

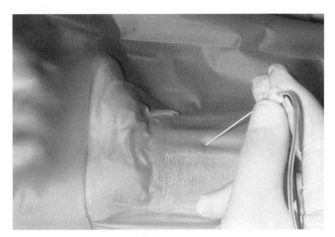

FIG. 25.

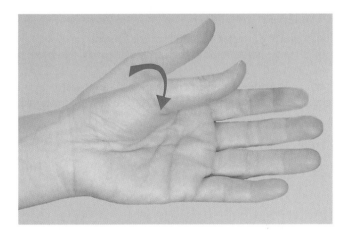

FIG. 26.

**Radial Nerve**

Block of the radial nerve at the wrist produces a field block of the superficial terminal branches because the nerve passes in a variable manner over the radial side of the wrist. The radial nerve branches are proximal to the anatomic snuffbox and should be blocked in a fan-shaped fashion without the use of a nerve stimulator **(Fig. 27)**.

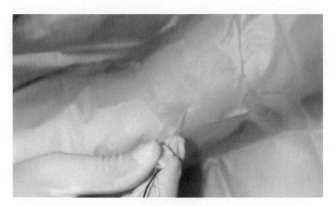

**FIG. 27.**

**TIPS**

1. These blocks preserve motor function of the fingers.
2. The use of a nerve stimulator is helpful to identify the median and the ulnar nerves.
3. The proper localization of these nerves allows the operator to minimize the volume of local anesthetic to be injected and reduce any theoretic risks of nerve compression.

# D. Digital Sheath Block

## Marcos V. Masson

**Patient Position:** The patient's hand is supinated.
**Needle Size:** 25-gauge, 2.5-cm needle.
**Indications:** Transthecal blocks are indicated for short digital procedures, especially in emergency situations.
**Volume:** 3 ml per digit.
**Anatomic Landmarks:** The anesthetic solution is injected into the space between the digital sheath and flexor tendon **(Fig. 28)**.

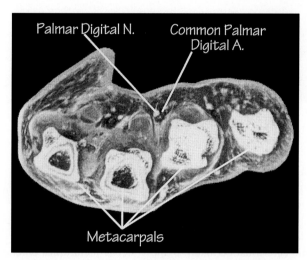

**FIG. 28.**

**Techniques and Approach:** With the hand in full supination, the patient is asked to extend and flex his or her fingers gently. The operator palpates the flexor tendon as it glides over the protuberance of the metacarpal head, then marks it with a skin pencil. The skin is penetrated at a 45-degree angle at the level of the distal skin crease of the palm just proximal to the metacarpophalangeal joint **(Fig. 29)**. Resistance is felt as the

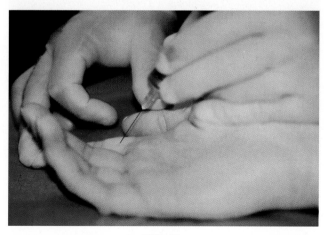

**FIG. 29.**

needle penetrates the flexor tendon sheath. The needle is then withdrawn slightly to sit above the tendon, at which point the local anesthetic solution is injected with the operator's index finger pressing down on the flexor tendon proximal to the metacarpophalangeal joint crease to prevent proximal flow of the local anesthetic solution **(Fig. 30)**. The bulging of the flexor tendon can be felt as the local anesthetic solution flows freely. Pressure is applied at the injection site for 3 or 4 minutes.

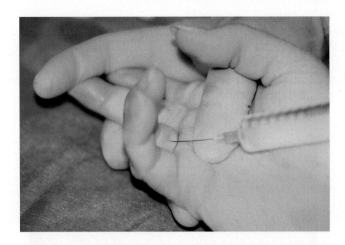

**FIG. 30.**

**TIPS**

1. Lidocaine 1% is the local anesthetic of choice.
2. When anesthetic solution is injected, the patient may experience a feeling of finger expansion **(Fig. 31)**.
3. This block produces analgesia distal to the palmar-digital crease that is more intense on the palmar side than on the dorsal side.
4. Considerable care must be taken to apply sterile techniques when performing this block to avoid contamination of the flexor tendon sheath. In this regard, the hands of both the operator and the patient should be disinfected with povidone-iodine, then with alcohol.
5. The onset of anesthesia is rapid, within 3 to 4 minutes of injection.
6. Compared with the conventional distal nerve block technique, the risk of mechanical trauma to the neurovascular bundle is minimal with this technique.

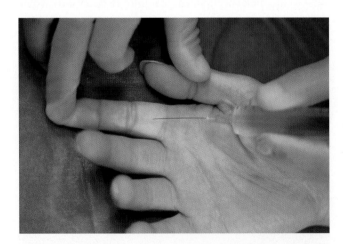

**FIG. 31.**

## SUGGESTED READINGS

Boulay G, Dupont X. Trans-thecal digital anesthesia in a case of section of the flexor tendon sheath. *Ann Fr Anesth Reanim* 1995;14:310.

Chiu DT. Transthecal digital block: flexor tendon sheath used for anesthetic infusion. *J Hand Surg* 1990;15:471–477.

Chevaleraud E, Ragot JM, Brunelle E, Dumontier C, Brunelli F. Local anesthesia of the finger through the flexor tendon sheath. *Ann Fr Anesth Reanim* 1993;12:237–240.

Chevaleraud E. Digital local anesthesia through the flexor sheath. *Cah Anesthesiol* 1993;41: 647–648.

Haribson S. Transthecal digital block: flexor tendon sheath used for anaesthetic infusion. *J Hand Surg* 1991;16:957.

Low CK, Vartany A, Diao E. Comparison of transthecal and subcutaneous single-injection digital block techniques in cadaver hands. *J Hand Surg* 1997;22:897–900.

Morrison WG. Transthecal digital block. *Arch Emerg Med* 1993;10:35–38.

Morros C, Perez D, Raurell A, Rodriquez JE. Digital anaesthesia through the flexor tendon sheath at the palmar level. *Int Orthop* 1993;17:273–274.

# 9

# General Considerations for Lower Extremity Blocks

Jacques E. Chelly

Lower extremity blocks, alone or in combination with general anesthesia, represent an interesting alternative to general anesthesia, spinal, and epidural anesthesia. Contrary to common belief, lower extremity blocks are not difficult to perform. With the exception of blocks performed for foot surgery, the nerves are often blocked higher than their terminal divisions. This produces extended motor and sensory blocks that often exceed surgical requirements. Most lower extremity blocks are performed using a nerve stimulator. In contrast to the endless discussion about the advantages and disadvantages of using a nerve stimulator, paresthesia, or a transarterial approach for upper extremity blocks, there is a clear consensus favoring the use of nerve stimulators for lower extremity blocks.

## ANATOMIC CONSIDERATIONS

Innervation of the lower extremity involves nerve roots L1 to S3 **(Fig. 1)**.

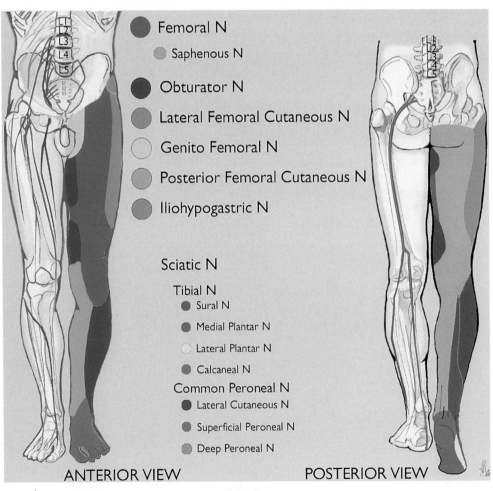

**FIG. 1.**

## Nerves of the Sciatic Plexus

The sciatic plexus comprises anterior branches of the ventral rami of the fourth and fifth lumbar nerves, as well as the first, second, and third sacral roots through the lumbosacral plexus (parasacral approach). Shortly afterward, it becomes the sciatic nerve, measuring approximately 1.5 to 2 cm in width and 0.3 to 0.5 cm in thickness, which makes it the largest nerve in the body. The sciatic nerve leaves the pelvis through the greater sciatic foramen and runs from the inferior border of the pyriformis muscles to the lower two-thirds of the femur, where it divides into two nerves, the tibial and common peroneal nerves. It provides innervation to the posterior aspect of the thigh through the posterior femoral cutaneous nerve. In the proximal part of its course, it remains on the posterior surface of the ischium covered by the gluteus maximus muscles (posterior approach). It leaves the pelvis and descends between the tuberosity of the ischium and the greater trochanter (Raj's anterior approach). In the distal part of its course, it runs posterior to the femur between the quadratus femoris and gluteus maximus muscles. Before running posterior to the femur below the ischial tuberosity and immediately below the lesser trochanter, the sciatic nerve travels for a short distance inferior and medial to the femur (Beck's or Chelly's anterior approach). Other anatomic landmarks include gluteal arteries in the vicinity of the nerve and the relationship between the sciatic nerve and the femoral nerve in the case of an anterior approach. In the popliteal fossa, the tibial nerve runs downward into the lower leg. The common peroneal nerve runs laterally along the medial aspect of the biceps femoris muscle. It enters the leg behind the head of the fibula. Before entering the longus muscle, it divides into the deep and superficial peroneal nerves. The common peroneal nerve provides motor and sensory innervation to the knee joint and the posterior and lateral aspect of the calf. The deep peroneal nerve runs down at the anterior aspect of the leg and medial to the tibial artery. At the ankle, it further divides into terminal branches. In the foot, the deep peroneal nerve runs medial to the callucis muscle and provides motor innervation to the tibialis anterior muscle and sensory innervation to the tarsal and metatarsal joints as well as the first and second interdigital space. The superficial peroneal nerve travels in the leg by the extensor digitorum longus muscle and divides into terminal branches just above the ankle. It provides sensory innervation to the dorsum of the foot and toes. The tibial nerve runs down deep in the soleus muscle. At the ankle, it runs medially between the Achilles tendon and medial malleolus before it divides into the lateral and medial plantar nerves. These nerves provide motor and sensory innervation to the heel and medial side of the foot below the territory innervated by the saphenous nerve and above one of the sural nerves. The sural nerve is a terminal branch of the posterior tibial nerve. It runs behind the lateral malleolus and between the malleolus and Achilles tendon. It provides sensory innervation to the lower and posterior aspects of the leg, as well as to the lateral aspect of the foot above the territory innervated by the calcaneal nerve, another branch of the posterior tibial nerve, and below the territory innervated by lateral cutaneous nerve, a branch of the common peroneal nerve.

## Nerves of the Lumbar Plexus

The lumbar plexus includes anterior branches of the ventral rami of the second to fifth lumbar nerves, which are individualized as the femoral nerve (L2-4), the lateral femoral cutaneous nerve (L2-3), the obturator nerve (L3-4), the genitofemoral nerve (L1-2), as well as the iliohypogastric and inguinal nerves (L1). Initially, the nerves lie in fascia anteriorly between the psoas and the quadratus lumborum muscle. The lateral femoral cutaneous, femoral, and obturator nerves lie in the pelvis on the iliacus muscle. They enter the thigh posterior to the inguinal ligament, with the lateral femoral nerve in close proximity to the anterior spinal crest spine, the femoral nerve in the middle between the anterior crest spine and the pubic tubercle, and the obturator nerve in a medial position and close to the pubic tubercle. The femoral nerve exits the inguinal ligament posterolateral to the femoral artery. It provides motor and sensory innervation to most of the anterior thigh and knee. The lateral femoral cutaneous nerve lies below the fascia lata after crossing the sartorius muscle at its origin, and immediately divides into anterior and posterior branches. The anterior branch supplies sensory innervation to the anterolateral aspect of the thigh, whereas the posterior branch supplies sensory innervation to the lateral and medial aspect of the thigh. The obturator nerve enters the obturator canal anterior to the obturator vessels in the canal and divides into posterior and anterior branches. The anterior branch supplies the anterior adductor muscle and sensory innervation to the hip as well as the medial aspect of the thigh below the territory innervated by the genitofemoral nerve. Finally, the saphenous nerve, which represents the main branch of the femoral nerve, originates above the knee and travels subcutaneously behind the medial femoral condyle. This nerve provides sensory innervation to the medial aspect of the leg, ankle, and a portion of the foot.

**Table 9.1.** *Peripheral nerve block techniques for common lower limb operations*

| Surgical Procedure | Peripheral Nerve Blocks | Remarks |
|---|---|---|
| Hip surgery | Lumbar plexus block or 3-in-1 block | Surgical and postoperative pain control. |
| Femur fractures | Lumbar plexus block or 3-in-1 block | Excellent analgesic technique for non-displaced closed reduction of the femur fracture. |
| Quadriceps muscle biopsy | 3-in-1 block | Lateral cutaneous nerve of the thigh block may be adequate for skin biopsy or skin graft of the lateral thigh. |
| Above knee amputation | Lumbar plexus block or 3-in-1 block and sciatic nerve block | Lumbar plexus block is preferred over the 3-in-1 block, since it is a more reliable approach to the obturator and lateral femoral cutaneous nerve block. |
| Knee arthroscopy Diagnostic Procedure | Lumbar plexus block or 3-in-1 block combined with the sciatic nerve block | Use lidocaine or chloroprocaine. A sciatic nerve block may also be needed when the operation involves the posterior part of the knee joint. |
| Total knee replacement Total hip replacement | Continuous lumbar plexus block or 3-in-1 block combined with single injection sciatic nerve | Narcotic (morphine, PRN, demerol) and/or anti-inflammatory (toradol may be needed to cover the postoperative posterior aspect of the knee). |
| Below knee amputation | Sciatic nerve block Popliteal fossa or above | The femoral nerve block is also needed to achieve anesthesia of the medial part of the lower leg, especially for the sciatic territory (total knee replacement). |
| Ankle surgery ORIF Ankle arthroscopy Achilles tendon repair | Sciatic nerve block Popliteal fossa or above | The femoral or saphenous nerve block is also needed to achieve anesthesia of the medial aspect of ankle. |
| Foot Surgery Bunionectomy Transmetatarsal Amputation Wound debridement | Ankle block or Popliteal block | When the popliteal block is used, the saphenous block may also be required for surgery involving the medial part of the foot. |
| Long saphenous vein stripping | Femoral nerve block | The genitofemoral nerve block is also required for proximal skin incision. |
| Short saphenous vein stripping | Sciatic nerve block above the popliteal fossa | Posterior cutaneous nerve of the thigh block is also required. |

## APPROACHES TO LOWER EXTREMITY BLOCKS

Lower extremity blocks can be performed with the patient in various positions (lateral, prone, or supine). Because lower extremity surgery usually requires a combination of blocks and because mobilization of the patient may be difficult or painful (e.g., arthritis, trauma), the choice of technique may be dictated by the need to limit mobilization of the patient. For surgery at the knee requiring sciatic and femoral blocks in a trauma patient who cannot be mobilized, anterior approaches to these two nerves are indicated. In contrast, when the patient can assume a prone or lateral position, a parasacral or posterior approach to the sciatic nerve combined with a lumbar plexus approach is possible.

Some consideration should also be given to the choice of the block according to the associated surgical requirements. For example, placement of the tourniquet at the thigh or the calf necessitates a lumbar plexus or 3-in-1 block or a saphenous nerve block, respectively. Although the arthroscopic knee diagnostic procedure requires only a 3-in-1 or femoral nerve block, any knee arthroscopic procedure involving the anterior aspect of the knee also requires block of the sciatic nerve. Surgery above the knee is usually performed using a parasacral, posterior, anterior, and popliteal approach to the sciatic nerve. A popliteal approach seems to be the approach of choice for surgery below the knee. As far as knee surgery is concerned, any block performed above the knee is appropriate. Finally, an overall block of the foot can be accomplished by an ankle block or a combined popliteal and saphenous or femoral block. The advantage of the latter approach is more prolonged analgesia, which is especially attractive for postoperative pain control. However, selective blocks are also being used for specific locations **(Table 1)**.

## SURGICAL INDICATIONS FOR LOWER EXTREMITY NERVE BLOCKS

Lower extremity blocks may be helpful in trauma, orthopedic and vascular surgeries, and radiographic procedures. However, careful considerations should be given to the relative position of nerves vis a vis to the bones, especially when there is displacement.

### Trauma

Patients with trauma to the lower extremity may greatly benefit from blocks for pain control. In this type of situation, the block often needs to be performed with the patient in a supine position.

### Vascular Surgery

For surgeries related to vascular diseases involving the lower extremities (below-knee amputation, debridement, and skin grafting), femoropopliteal and tibial arterial reconstruction, as well as for the removal of varices, the use of lower extremity blocks is of special interest. Because of their lack of effects on the cardiovascular system, their use remains limited. In this regard, it is important to recognize that a sciatic nerve block is unnecessary for removing the internal saphenous veins. A femoral block is adequate. Finally, anticoagulant therapy is a contraindication to sciatic nerve block.

### Orthopedic Surgery

There are a number of indications for nerve blocks in orthopedic surgery of the lower extremity **(Table 1; Fig. 2)**.

### Hip

It is unclear whether a peripheral nerve block can adequately provide pain control for hip surgery. The use of a continuous lumbar plexus or 3-in-1 block is an interesting option for postoperative pain control after total hip replacement.

# Foot Procedures

| | Plantar | Saphenous | Deep Peroneal | Peroneal Superficial | Sural |
|---|---|---|---|---|---|
| Hallux valgus | + | +/- | + | + | |
| Hallux rigidus | + | +/- | + | + | |
| 1st Toe | + | | + | + | |
| 2nd Toe | + | | + | + | |
| 3rd Toe | + | | | + | |
| 4th Toe | + | | | + | |
| 5th Toe | + | | | | + |
| Heel | + | | | | |

FIG. 2. Foot Procedures (figure prepared by Philippe Macaire, M.D.).

## Knee

Although diagnostic knee arthroscopy can be performed under local anesthesia or a femoral or, better, a 3-in-1 block, a combination of a 3-in-1 and a sciatic nerve block is necessary to satisfy the requirements of any surgery at the knee. For a total knee replacement, a continuous 3-in-1 block and a single-injection sciatic nerve block is the preferred choice. Thus, the main immediate postoperative complication after a total knee replacement is the occurrence of a compression syndrome in the posterior compartment resulting in sciatic nerve compression. This technique does not compromise the early diagnosis of compression syndrome. After surgery, analgesic (morphine PRN) or anti-inflammatory drugs (toradol) are used to provide pain control in the sciatic territory. The use of a continuous 3-in-1 block also allows for an early start of physical therapy.

## Below the Knee

Sciatic and femoral or saphenous blocks are required to satisfy surgical requirements in this territory. Sciatic nerve blocks using single injection or continuous infusions are also attractive for pain control of tibial fractures (rods, placement of external or internal fixation).

## Foot

Although ankle blocks represent a classical approach to surgical and postoperative analgesia, popliteal sciatic nerve blocks associated with saphenous nerve blocks when necessary are gaining acceptance for foot surgery. Selective blocks of the sciatic nerve branches also represent an alternative to limit the extent of motor block.

## CHARACTERISTICS OF LOWER EXTREMITY BLOCKS

Doppler ultrasound can be used to facilitate identification of the superior gluteal artery, and fluoroscopy has been used to identify the dorsal surface of the ischium in patients in a prone position. Both methods remain anecdotal.

Except in the popliteal fossa, the sciatic nerve block has the longest onset and duration of peripheral blocks commonly performed by anesthesiologists. A minimum of 10 to 20 minutes, and in most cases, 30 minutes, is required to allow a complete block. This delay can be reduced by the addition of bicarbonates and epinephrine or by using a higher concentration of local anesthetic solution. However, such a long onset needs to be taken into consideration when defining the anesthesia strategy. On the other hand, sciatic nerve blocks often last more than 12 hours, and up to 16 hours when performed with bupivacaine and ropivacaine. Such a persistent block favors the use of a single injection, rather than continuous infusion. This contrasts with a femoral block that only requires 5 to 10 minutes or less, depending on the local anesthetic solution. Furthermore, the placement of a catheter is indicated mainly for patients requiring more than 24 hours of acute pain control.

Of the different popliteal approaches, the one in the prone position is the easiest.

Various local anesthetics in various concentrations have been used to block the sciatic and femoral nerve. Except for ankle blocks, we favor the use of 1.5% lidocaine or mepivacaine with epinephrine and 0.75% ropivacaine. The total volume of local anesthetic solution required to block a lower extremity is often 60 ml (sciatic and 3-in-1 blocks). In this regard, the better safety profile of ropivacaine compared to bupivacaine makes ropivacaine especially attractive when multiple lower extremity blocks are performed. However, the use of local anesthetics with shorter half-lives may also be indicated to favor early discharge when recovery of motor function is required for discharge. Thus, the duration of a diagnostic knee arthroscopy, which may vary from 10 to 45 minutes, may justify the use of either lidocaine or mepivacaine alone.

## SUGGESTED READINGS

Beck GP. Anterior approach to sciatic nerve block. *Anesthesiology* 1963;24:222–224.

Capellino A, Jokl P, Ruwe PA. Regional anesthesia in knee arthroscopy: a new technique involving femoral and sciatic nerve blocks in knee arthroscopy. *Arthroscopy* 1996;12:120–123.

Chelly JE, Greger J, Howard G. Simple interior approach for sciatic blockade. *Reg Anesth* 1997;22:114(abst).

Coventry DM, Todd JG. Alkalinization of bupivacaine for sciatic nerve blockade. *Anesthesia* 1989; 44:467–470.

Davies MJ, McGlade DP. One hundred sciatic nerve blocks: a comparison of localisation techniques. *Anaesth Intensive Care* 1993;21:76–78.

Giordano JM, Morales GA, Trout HH, DePalma RG. Regional nerve block for femoropopliteal and tibial arterial reconstructions. *Vascular Surgery* 1986;4:351–354.

Ichiyanagi K. Sciatic nerve block: lateral approach with patient supine. *Anesthesiology* 1959;20: 601–604.

Labat G. *Regional anaesthesia: its technique and clinical applications*, 2nd ed. Philadelphia: WB Saunders, 1930:330.

Mansour NY. Re-evaluating the sciatic nerve block: another landmark for consideration. *Reg Anesth* 1993;18:322–323.

Raj PP, Parks RI, Watson TD, Jenkins MT. A new single-position supine approach to sciatic-femoral nerve block. *Anesth Analg* 1975;54:489–493.

Tagariello V, Bertini L, Mancini S, et al. Sciatic and femoral nerve block with ropivacaine. *Reg Anesth and Pain Med* 1998;23S:18.

Winnie AP, Ramamurthy S, Durrani Z. The inguinal paravascular technique of lumbar plexus anesthesia: the 3-in-1 block. *Anesth Analg* 1973;52:989–996.

Winne AP. Regional anaesthesia. *Surg Clin North Am* 1975;54:861–892.

# 10

# Sciatic Nerve Blocks

# A. Parasacral Approach

## Gary F. Morris and Jacques E. Chelly

**Patient Position:** The patient is positioned laterally with the operative limb uppermost. The hip and knee are slightly flexed to facilitate patient comfort.

**Indications:** Unilateral lower extremity surgery, including posterior aspect of the leg, the knee, and below the knee.

**Needle size:** 21-gauge, 100-mm b-beveled Stimuplex insulated needle (B. Braun/McGaw Medical, Inc., Bethlehem, PA).

**Volume:** 30 ml.

**Anatomic Landmarks:** The sacral plexus consists of nerve fibers originating from the L4 to S3 nerve roots. These nerve roots travel within the pelvis anterior to the ischial bone and the piriformis muscle. They then coalesce to form the common peroneal, tibial, posterior femoral cutaneous, inferior gluteal, and superior gluteal nerves just before exiting the pelvis through the greater sciatic notch immediately caudal to the piriformis muscle. In addition to the components of the sciatic nerve, the sacral plexus also gives rise to the pudendal nerve. The pelvic splanchnic nerves (S2-4), the terminal portion of the sympathetic trunk, and the inferior hypogastric plexus all lie in close proximity to the elements of the sacral plexus.

**Approach and Technique:** The posterior superior iliac spine is identified and a line is constructed between that point and the ischial tuberosity **(Fig. 1)**. At a point approximately 3 fingerbreadths (6 cm) from the posterior superior iliac spine, a 100-mm b-beveled insulated Stimuplex needle (B. Braun/McGaw Medical, Inc., Bethlehem, PA), connected to a nerve stimulator set to deliver 2 mA, is inserted and advanced in a sagittal plane **(Fig. 2)**. The needle is walked off the contour of the greater sciatic notch into the pelvis. A brisk motor response at the ankle is sought with the aid of a peripheral nerve stimulator. Once a motor response is elicited at 0.2 mA (Digistim II, Neurotechnology, Houston, TX), 30 ml of local anesthetic is injected **(Figs. 3 to 7)**.

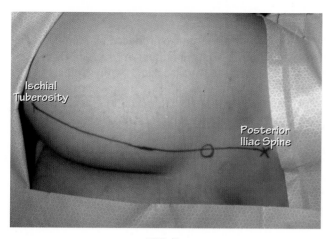

**FIG. 1.**

Ischial Tuberosity

Posterior Iliac Spine

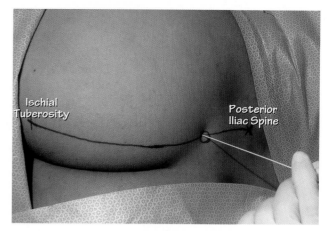

**FIG. 2.**

Ischial Tuberosity

Posterior Iliac Spine

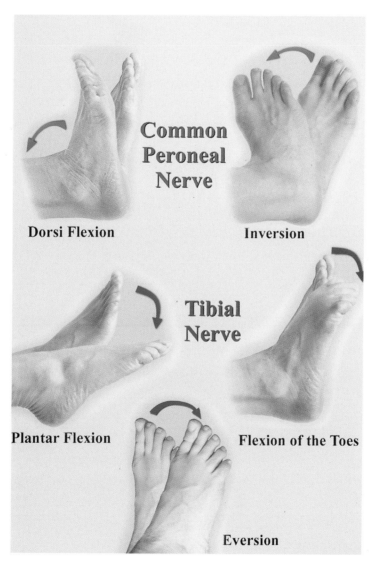

**Common Peroneal Nerve**

Dorsi Flexion

Inversion

**Tibial Nerve**

Plantar Flexion

Flexion of the Toes

Eversion

**FIG. 3.**

## TIPS

1. The onset rate is independent of the type of response produced by stimulation by the sciatic nerve (e.g., plantar flexion [tibial] or dorsiflexion [peroneal]).
2. The parasacral sciatic approach is commonly associated with a block of the pudendal and obturator nerves.

## SUGGESTED READINGS

Bruelle P, Cuvillon P, Ripart J, Eledjam JJ. Sciatic nerve block: parasacral approach. *Regional Anesthesia and Pain Med* 1998;23:78.

Mansour NY, Bennetts. An observational study of combined continuous lumbar plexus and single-shot sciatic nerve blocks for post-knee surgery analgesia. *Reg Anesth* 1996;21:287–291.

Morris GF, Lang SA, Dust WN, Van der Wal M. The parasacral sciatic nerve block. *Reg Anesth* 1997;22:223–228.

# B. Posterior Approach

## Daneshvari Solanki

**Patient Position:** The patient is placed in a lateral position with the operative site up and the knee flexed at 90 degrees. The knee of the uppermost extremity rests on the knee of the bottom leg.

**Indication:** Unilateral lower extremity surgery.

**Needle size:** 21-gauge, 100-mm b-beveled Stimuplex insulated needle (B. Braun/McGaw Medical, Inc., Bethlehem, PA).

**Volume:** 15 to 25 ml of local anesthetic.

**Anatomic Landmarks:** The sciatic nerve is formed by the inferior divisions of the L4, L5, S1, S2, and S3 nerves **(Fig. 4)**. It exits the pelvis through the greater sciatic notch and passes between the greater trochanter and the ischial tuberosity. Sciatic innervation is shown in **Fig. 5**.

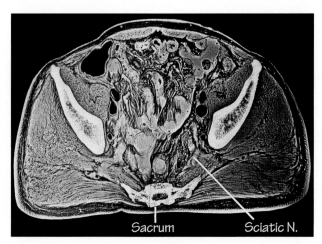

FIG. 4.

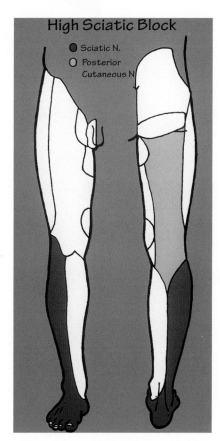

FIG. 5.

**Approach and Technique:** The highest point of the greater trochanter is identified and marked. A line is drawn from this point to the posterior superior iliac spine. Another line is drawn from the greater trochanter to the sacral hiatus. A line perpendicular to the midpoint of the greater trochanter to the posterior iliac spine line is drawn. The intersection of this line with the grater trochanter to the sacral hiatus line represents the point of insertion of the needle **(Fig. 6)**. The b-beveled insulated

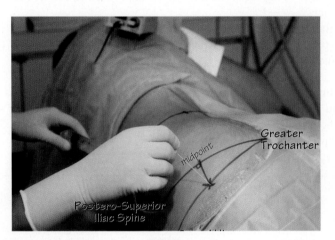

**FIG. 6.**

needle is introduced through this point perpendicular to all planes. Nerve stimulator current is set at 5 mA. If the bone is contacted, the needle must be withdrawn and directed caudally. Contraction of gastrocnemius (plantar flexion of the foot) or contraction of the tibialis anterior (dorsiflexion of the foot) indicates proximity to the sciatic nerve **(Fig. 7)**. Current is then decreased to 0.5 mA. If the response is still present, 15 to 20 ml of local anesthetic is injected after a negative aspiration.

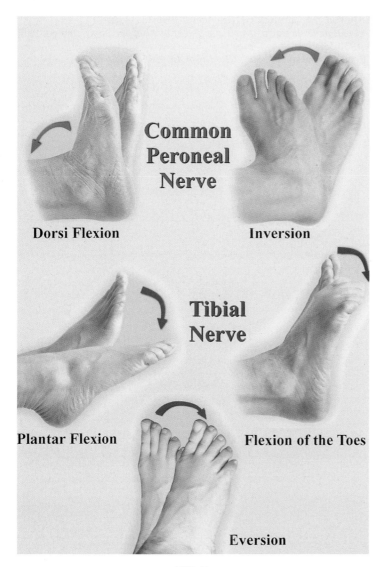

**FIG. 7.**

## TIPS

1. Positioning of the patient as described previously is vital to establish the anatomic landmarks.
2. If bone is contacted when the needle is placed perpendicular to all planes, it is probably on the greater sciatic notch. The needle must be redirected caudally.

## SUGGESTED READINGS

Hahn M, McQuillan PM, Sheplock GJ. *Reg Anesth* 1996;121–131.

Labat G. *Regional anaesthesia: its technique and clinical applications*, 2nd ed. Philadelphia: WB Saunders, 1930:330.

Winnie AP. Regional anaesthesia. *Surg Clin North Am* 1975;54:861–892.

# C. Anterior Approach

## Jacques E. Chelly

**Patient Position:** The patient remains in the supine position with the lower extremity in the neutral position.

**Indications:** Surgery of the knee and below. Pain relief for trauma of the lower extremity.

**Needle Size:** 20-gauge, 150-mm b-beveled Stimuplex insulated needle (E. Braun/McGaw Medical, Inc., Bethlehem, PA).

**Volume:** 20 to 30 ml.

**Anatomic Landmarks:** Anterior iliac spine and superior border of the pubic tubercle. The sciatic nerve passes from the lower border of the gluteus maximus, runs down the thigh, lying first medial to the femur and then crossing on the posterior medial aspect of the femur **(Figs. 8,9).**

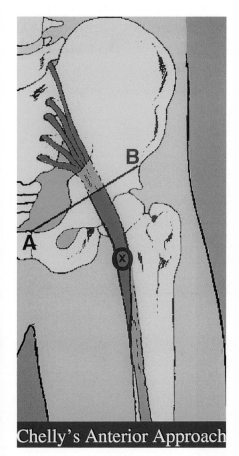

Chelly's Anterior Approach

**FIG. 8.**

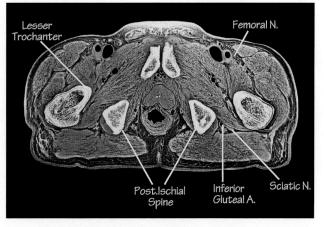

**FIG. 9.**

**Approach and Technique:** A sacropubic line is drawn between the anterior iliac spine and the superior angle of the pubic tubercle. At its midpoint, a perpendicular line is drawn. The site of introduction of the needle is 8 cm from the top of this perpendicular line **(Figs. 10 to 12).** The 150-mm b-beveled insulated Stimuplex needle (E. Braun/McGaw Medical, Inc., Bethlehem, PA), connected to a nerve stimulator set to

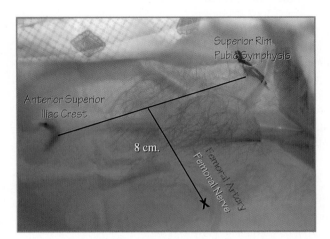

**FIG. 10.**

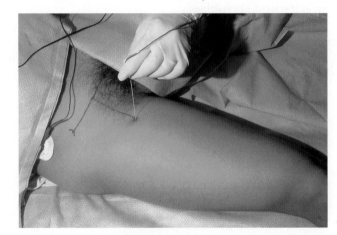

**FIG. 11.**

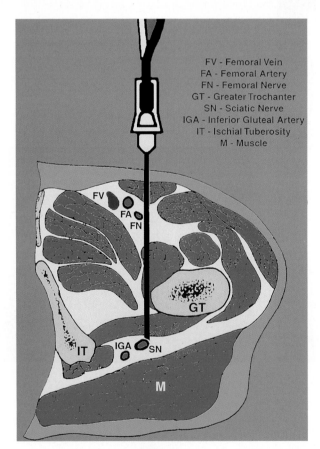

FV - Femoral Vein
FA - Femoral Artery
FN - Femoral Nerve
GT - Greater Trochanter
SN - Sciatic Nerve
IGA - Inferior Gluteal Artery
IT - Ischial Tuberosity
M - Muscle

**FIG. 12.**

deliver 1.5 mA, is introduced vertically. If the femur is contacted, the needle is removed and introduced 1.5 to 2 cm medially. Stimulation of the sciatic nerve is usually obtained at a depth of 10 to 12 cm. It produces plantar or dorsal flexion or eversion or incision of the foot and flexion of the toes **(Fig. 13)**.

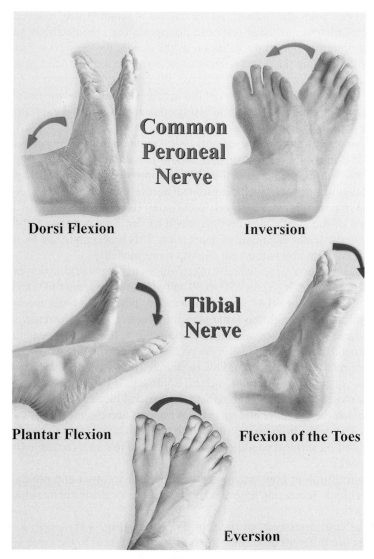

Common Peroneal Nerve

Dorsi Flexion          Inversion

Tibial Nerve

Plantar Flexion          Flexion of the Toes

Eversion

**FIG. 13.**

## TIPS

1. In this approach, the nerve stimulator has a dual function. First, it helps prevent damage to the femoral nerve during the first 5 cm of needle introduction, and second, it helps to localize the sciatic nerve. As for any other block, the nerve stimulator is first set at 1.5 mA after the needle passes the skin. Within 2 to 5 cm of depth, a contraction of the quadriceps (femoral nerve) or the medial aspect of the thigh (obturator nerve) appears. At this point, the intensity of the current is progressively reduced to 1 mA or less to verify that the muscular response disappears (i.e., the needle is not facing the femoral or obturator nerve). Progression of the needle for the next 1.5 cm is accomplished while keeping the nerve stimulator at the same setting. After passing through the territory of the femoral/obturator nerve, the current is increased to its original 5-mA value. If during the introduction of the needle it is found that the needle is directly on the femoral or obturator nerve, the insulated needle is directed away from the nerve before continuing with any further advancement.

2. Except for morbidly obese patients (>400 pounds), it is rarely necessary to introduce the 150-mm b-beveled insulated needle more than 12 cm to find the sciatic nerve. In most cases, the nerve is found at an approximate depth of 10 to 12 cm.

3. Introduction of a b-beveled insulated needle through the quadriceps gives an impression of going through relatively soft tissue. However, at a depth of 10 to 12 cm, introduction of the needle may become much harder. This is a sign that the needle is very close to the femur and requires redirection. This is accomplished by removing the needle at least 2 cm and redirecting slightly more medially.

4. The sciatic nerve block usually takes longer to set up than upper extremity and femoral nerve blocks. It requires 20 to 30 minutes or even longer to take effect.

5. Using the anterior sciatic approach, it is also possible to block the more superficial femoral nerve through the same skin introduction point. However, to avoid any risk of damage with the b-beveled insulated needle to the femoral or obturator nerve, we recommend blocking the sciatic nerve and then proceeding to block the femoral nerve while retracting the needle. This technique offers the advantage of sticking the patient only once. However, with such an approach, it is not possible to do a 3-in-1 block. The closer to the inguinal ligament the femoral block is performed, the easier it is also to block the obturator and superficial femoral nerves, because of their anatomic proximity. The decision to use one approach rather than the other to block the femoral nerve is based on surgical conditions and the need to use a tourniquet (which requires a 3-in-1 block).

6. Alkalinization of bupivacaine reduces the time to onset and prolongs the duration of this block. Increasing the concentration of the local anesthetic solution has similar effects.

7. Beck first described an anterior approach **(Fig. 14)**. Chelly's and Beck's approaches use different anatomic landmarks but both lead to the same site **(Fig. 15)**.

8. Finally, another anterior approach has been described by Raj **(Fig. 16)**. Anatomical landmarks include the ischial tuberosity and the greater trochanter. The 150 mm insulated b-beveled needle is introduced in the middle, perpendicular to the skin.

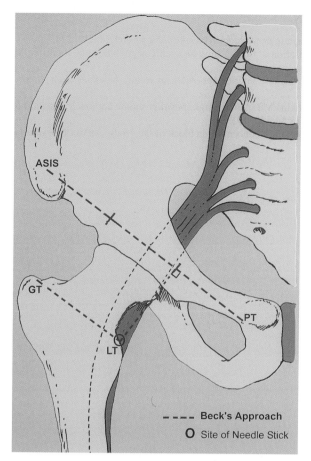

FIG. 14.

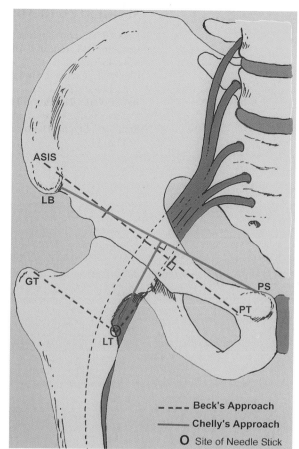

FIG. 15.

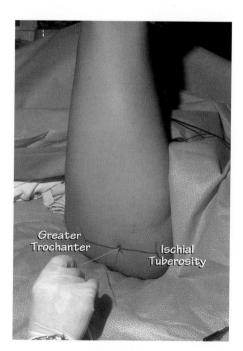

FIG. 16.

## SUGGESTED READINGS

Beck GP. Anterior approach to sciatic nerve block. *Anesthesiology* 1963;24:222–224.

Coventry DM, Todd JG. Alkalinisation of bupivacaine for sciatic nerve blockade. *Anaesthesia* 1989; 44:467–470.

Chelly JE, Greger J, Howard G. Simple interior approach for sciatic blockade. *Reg Anesth* 1997; 22:114(abst).

Raj PP, Parks RI, Watson TD, Jenkins MT. A new single-position supine approach to sciatic-femoral nerve block. *Anesth Analg* 1975;54:489–493.

Smith BE, Siggins D. Low volume, high concentration block of the sciatic nerve. *Anaesthesia* 1988; 43:8–11.

# D. Posterior Popliteal Approach

Jacques E. Chelly

**Patient Position:** The patient is placed in the lateral position with the operative side up, or in the prone position. The upper leg to be blocked should be straight or slightly flexed.

**Indications:** Surgery at and below the knee. This block is usually combined with the femoral or saphenous nerve block to obtain complete anesthesia below the knee.

**Needle size:** 21-gauge, 100-mm b-beveled Stimuplex insulated needle (B. Braun/ McGaw Medical, Inc., Bethlehem, PA).

**Volume:** 10 to 15 ml.

**Anatomic Landmarks:** The sciatic nerve splits into the common peroneal and tibial nerves just proximal to the knee **(Fig. 17).** To get a complete lower extremity block, the sciatic nerve must be blocked before its division. The sciatic nerve innervation at the popliteal fossa is shown in **Fig. 18.**

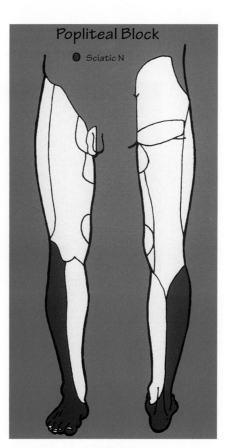

Popliteal Block

Sciatic N

**FIG.18.**

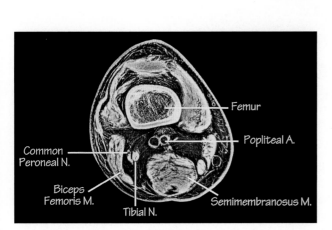

Femur

Popliteal A.

Common Peroneal N.

Biceps Femoris M.

Tibial N.

Semimembranosus M.

**FIG. 17.**

**Approach and Technique:** A line is drawn across the midpopliteal fossa crease. A midpoint perpendicular line is then extended 5 cm cephalad. The 100-mm b-beveled insulated Stimuplex needle (B. Braun/McGaw Medical, Inc., Bethlehem, PA), connected to a nerve stimulator set to deliver 1.5 mA, is introduced 1 cm lateral to the perpendicular line and angled at 45 degrees from the skin in a cephalad direction **(Figs. 19 to 21).** The needle is advanced 2 to 5 cm until the sciatic nerve is stimulated. The stimulation of the sciatic nerve usually results in plantar flexion or flexion of the toes.

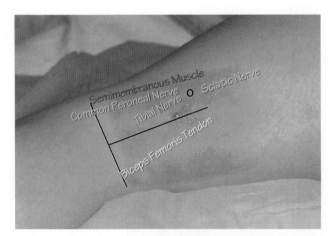

FIG. 19.

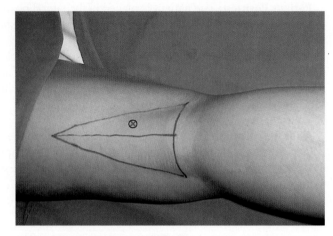

FIG. 20.

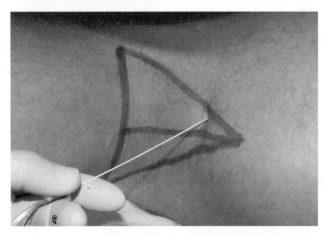

FIG. 21.

## TIPS

1. It is easier to find the sciatic nerve with the patient in the prone position.
2. Saphenous nerve block is often required to complement the sciatic block, especially for surgery at or below the knee. For this purpose, a 25-gauge 25-mm needle is introduced subcutaneously between the head of the tibia and the middle of the muscle. Ten milliliters of local anesthetic solution is injected at a depth of 3 cm. This injection produces anesthesia of the medial aspect of the leg.

## SUGGESTED READING

Comfort VK, Lang SA, Yip RW. Saphenous nerve anaesthesia: a nerve stimulator technique. *Can J Anaesth* 1996;43:852–857.

# E. Lateral Popliteal Approach

Jerry D. Vloka and Admir Hadžić

**Patient Position:** Supine.

**Indications:** Surgery below the knee.

**Needle:** 21-gauge, 100-mm b-beveled insulated needle (B. Braun/McGaw Medical, Inc., Bethlehem, PA).

**Volume:** 40 ml.

**Anatomic Landmarks:** Lateral femoral epicondyle, groove between biceps femoris and vastus lateralis muscles.

**Approach and Technique:** The block is performed with the patient in the supine position, with the leg extended at the knee joint. The long axis of the foot is positioned at a 90-degree angle relative to the table. A 100-mm b-beveled insulated needle (B. Braun/McGaw Medical, Inc., Bethlehem, PA), attached to a low-output nerve stimulator, is inserted in a horizontal plane 7 cm cephalad to the most prominent point of the lateral femoral epicondyle **(Fig. 22).** The 100-mm needle connected to a nerve stimulator set to deliver 1 mA, is inserted in the groove between the biceps femoris and the vastus lateralis muscles until the shaft of the femoral bone is contacted. Once the femoral bone is contacted, the needle is withdrawn to the skin, and redirected posteriorly at a 30-degree angle to the horizontal plane (Fig. 26). If the sciatic nerve is not stimulated, the needle is withdrawn to the skin and reinserted through the same skin puncture, first 5 to 10° anterior and then 5 to 10° posterior relative to the initial insertion (30-degree) plane. If these redirections do not result in nerve localization, the same technique is repeated through new skin punctures in 5-mm increments posterior to the initial insertion plane **(Fig. 23)**.

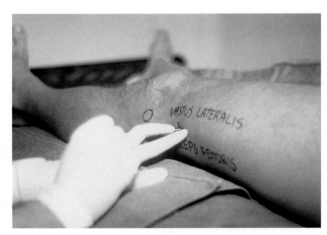

FIG. 22.

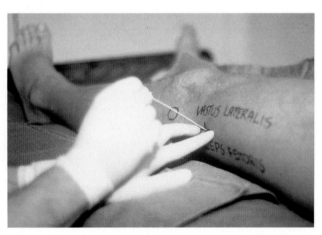

FIG. 23.

## TIPS

1. A fast onset and the most consistent results for surgical anesthesia are achieved when 40 ml or more of 1.5% alkalinized mepivacaine (1 mEq of $NaHCO_3$/30 ml) with 1:200,000 epinephrine is used.
2. Bupivacaine 0.25% to 0.375% with epinephrine is used for postoperative analgesia.
3. Plantar flexion (tibial nerve) or dorsal flexion (common peroneal nerve) of the foot or toes are signs of proper needle position.
4. Ideally, stimulation of the nerve is achieved using a current of 0.4 mA or less. When this is not possible (e.g., diabetic, elderly, or septic patients), stimulation of the division of the sciatic nerve that predominantly innervates the surgical area should be sought.
5. Supplementary block of the saphenous nerve (or femoral nerve) is required for surgery involving the medial aspect of the leg.

## SUGGESTED READINGS

Hadžić A, Vloka JD. A comparison of the posterior versus lateral approaches to the block of the sciatic nerve in the popliteal fossa. *Anesthesiology* 1988;88:1480–1486.

Vloka JD, Hadžić A, Kitain E, et al. Anatomic considerations for sciatic nerve block in the popliteal fossa through the lateral approach. *Reg Anesth* 1996;21:414–418.

# 11

# Femoral, Obturator, and Lateral Femoral Cutaneous Blocks

# A. Posterior Lumbar Plexus (Psoas) Block

## Daneshvari Solanki

**Patient Position:** The patient lies in a lateral position (Sim's position) with the operative side up.

**Indications:** Unilateral lower extremity surgery.

**Needle size:** 21-gauge, 100-mm b-beveled Stimuplex insulated needle (B. Braun/McGaw Medical, Inc., Bethlehem, PA).

**Volume:** 20 to 30 ml.

**Anatomic Landmarks:** The lumbar plexus originates from the ventral roots of the first four lumbar nerves **(Fig. 1)**. It lies within the psoas muscle, anterior to the transverse processes of the lumbar vertebrae. The plexus is triangular in shape. It is narrow at the superior portion but wider in the inferior portion.

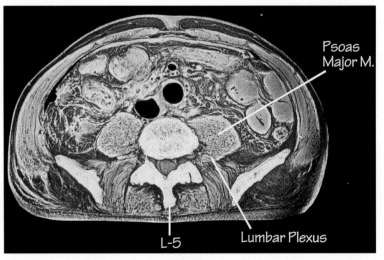

**FIG. 1.**

**Approach and Technique:** Spinous processes of the third, fourth, and fifth lumbar vertebrae are identified. A line is drawn through these points. This is the midline. The posterior superior iliac spine is identified. A line is drawn parallel to the midline, passing through this point. The distance between these two lines is 4.5 to 5 cm **(Fig. 2)**. The highest point of the iliac crest is identified. A line perpendicular to the other two lines is drawn from the point on the iliac crest. The intersection of the two latter lines represents the point of insertion of the needle. The 100-mm b-beveled insulated Stimuplex needle (B. Braun/McGaw Medical, Inc., Bethlehem, PA), connected to a nerve stimulator set to deliver 2 mA, is introduced (perpendicular to all planes) through this point and advanced until contact with the transverse process of L5. If the bone is not contacted, the needle must be withdrawn and directed 10 degrees cephalad until it is contacted. The needle is then advanced so that it slides underneath the bone. A loss of resistance is felt. The needle enters the psoas compartment **(Fig. 3)**. The nerve stimulator is kept at 2 mA, and contraction of the quadriceps muscle is sought. The current is turned down to 0.5 mA, and if contraction of the quadriceps is still present, 20 to 25 ml of local anesthetic is injected after a negative aspiration for blood or fluid, producing abolition of this response.

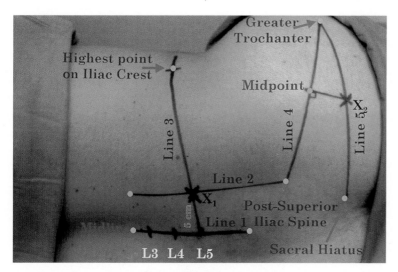

**FIG. 2.**

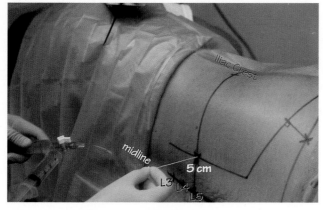

**FIG. 3.**

## TIPS

1. The lumbar plexus is usually at a depth of 7 to 8 cm.
2. Except for morbidly obese patients, it is rarely necessary to use a 150-mm insulated needle.
3. Any attempt to reach the lumbar plexus by a more medial approach may cause bilateral anesthesia due to epidural anesthesia, spinal anesthesia, or other mechanisms.
4. A needle inserted more than 6 cm away from the midline can completely miss the psoas major muscle.
5. Insertion of the needle more than 11 cm deep (if a 150-mm needle is used in normal patients) can result in retroperitoneal injection.
6. Inject 25 to 30 ml of local anesthetic at the lumbar plexus if the surgery is in the upper two-thirds of the lower extremity, and the remaining 15 ml at the sciatic region.
7. If the surgery is in the lower one-third of the extremity, inject 25 to 30 ml of local anesthetic at the sciatic region and 15 to 20 ml at the lumbar plexus.

## SUGGESTED READINGS

Chayen D, Nathan H, Chayen M. The psoas compartment block. *Anesthesiology* 1976;45:95–99.

Farny J, Drolet P, Girard M. Anatomy of the posterior approach to the lumbar plexus block. *Can J Anaesth* 1994;41:480–485.

Hahn M, McQuillan PM, Sheplock GJ. *Reg Anesth* 1996;121:131.

Winnie AP, Ramamurthy S, Durrani Z, Radonjic R. Plexus blocks for lower extremity surgery. *Anesthesiology Review* 1974;00:11–16.

# B. Fascia Iliacus Block

## Jeff J. Rockwell

**Patient Position:** The patient is placed supine, legs flat, with operative leg slightly abducted.

**Indications:** Used primarily for postoperative pain relief for anterior cruciate ligament repair and total knee replacements, but can be used for any surgery involving distribution of femoral, obturator, and lateral femoral cutaneous nerves.

**Needle:** 20-gauge, Arrow bullet-tip needle with 18-gauge catheter (Arrow International, Inc., Reading, PA).

**Volume:** 0.7 ml/kg body weight up to a maximum of 60 ml.

**Anatomic Landmarks:** The target nerves: femoral (dorsal L2-4), lateral femoral cutaneous (dorsal L2-3), and obturator (ventral L2-4) all run immediately posterior to the fascia iliacus during their initial course. The lateral femoral cutaneous is the first to emerge from the lateral border of the psoas muscle at about its midpoint. The obturator leaves the compartment next, from the medial boarder of the psoas muscle near the pelvic brim. The femoral nerve travels down the lateral margin of the psoas in the groove between the psoas and iliacus muscles. Local anesthesia, tracking proximally, within this compartment will contact the three target nerves. Fluoroscopy can track the solution of local anesthetic within the fascia iliacus compartment well above the pelvic brim (**Fig. 4**).

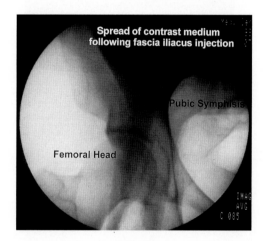

**FIG. 4.**

**Approach and Technique:** A line between the anterior superior iliac spine and symphysis pubis is drawn. This denotes the course of the inguinal ligament. Palpate the femoral pulse approximately 3 to 4 cm below the inguinal ligament. Needle placement is 1 fingerbreadth lateral to femoral pulse at this point. First, make a skin nick with 18-gauge sharp beveled needle (included in kit). Then place Arrow BP-01200 bullet-tip needle and catheter through skin nick. Aim cephalad at approximately 45 degrees from skin for placement beneath the inguinal canal. This is a two-pop loss of resistance technique. The first pop represents penetration of the fascia lata, after which firm resistance should be met. Applying firm pressure, a second pop places the needle and catheter beneath the fascia iliacus **(Fig. 5)**. Now flatten the angle slightly, advance another 1 cm, and slide the catheter off. It should advance easily to the hub. Attach the syringe and apply firm distal groin pressure to encourage proximal tracking of local anesthetic. Aspirate and inject the chosen local anesthetic incrementally. Then heparin lock and secure the catheter for postoperative reinjection.

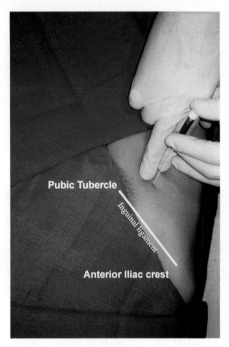

Pubic Tubercle

Inguinal ligament

Anterior Iliac crest

**FIG. 5.**

**TIPS**

1. This block is primarily for postoperative pain relief in knee surgeries. It is especially useful for anterior cruciate ligament repairs.
2. Be sure to trace the proximal route of the femoral artery and stay lateral to avoid arterial puncture.
3. The fascia iliacus is dense and the needle is blunt, so surprisingly firm pressure is often required for the second pop.
4. In thin patients, occasionally only one large pop is obtained.
5. Because of the pressure required to insert bullet-tipped needle, the block is placed with heavy sedation or after induction of general anesthesia. Bullet tip makes nerve damage unlikely.
6. Incremental injection with 0.20% to 0.25% ropivacaine with epinephrine allows detection of intravascular injection.
7. Catheters are left for reinjection before discharge home or that night if admission is planned.

8. Patients with hamstring tendon anterior cruciate ligament repair may have posterior discomfort. This can be relieved with oral narcotics, nonsteroidal anti-inflammatory drugs, or a single-injection sciatic block.
9. Keep in mind that the efficacy of this block depends on volume. The concentration of local anesthetic may need to be limited to avoid potential systemic toxicity. The addition of epinephrine may also help achieve this goal.

## SUGGESTED READINGS

Dalens B, Vanneuville G, Tanguy A. Comparison of the fascia iliac compartment block with the 3-in-1 block in children. *Anesth Analg* 1989;69:705–713.
Winnie AP, Ramamurthy S, Durrani Z. The inguinal paravascular technique of lumbar plexus anesthesia: the 3-in-1 block. *Anesth Analg* 1973;52:989–996.

# C. Femoral Block

## Jacques E. Chelly

**Patient Position:** Supine position.

**Indications:** Arthroscopy and surgery of the knee. Surgery above the knee is often combined with obturator and lateral femoral cutaneous nerve blocks (3-in-1 block). Surgery below the knee is combined with a 3-in-1 or saphenous nerve block (depending on surgical requirements and the position of the tourniquet) and a sciatic nerve block.

**Needle Size:** 24-gauge, 25-mm b-beveled Stimuplex insulated needle (B. Braun/McGaw Medical, Inc., Bethlehem, PA).

**Volume:** 15 to 20 ml.

**Anatomic Landmarks:** The femoral nerve is located just 1 to 2 cm lateral to the femoral artery below the inguinal ligament **(Figs. 6, 7).** Femoral nerve innervation is shown in **Fig. 8.**

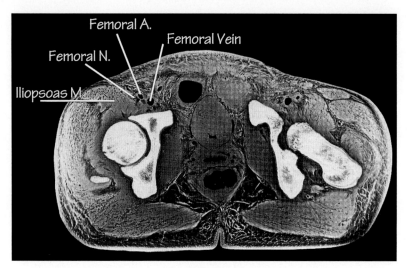

FIG. 6.

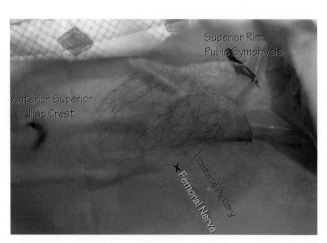

FIG. 7.

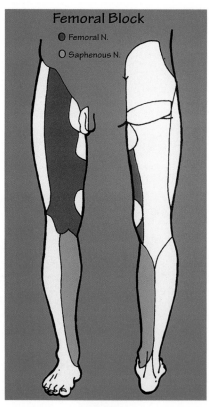

FIG. 8.

**Approach and Technique:** The femoral nerve is a relatively superficial nerve. It is usually found with a 25-mm b-beveled insulated Stimuplex needle (B. Braun/McGaw Medical, Inc., Bethlehem, PA) connected to a nerve stimulator set to deliver 1.5 mA **(Fig. 9)**. The needle is introduced perpendicular to the skin until stimulation of the nerve produces movements of the patella **(Fig. 10)**.

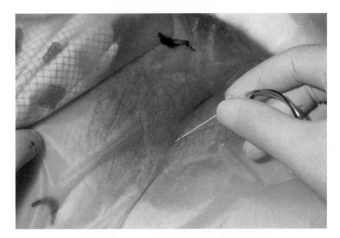

**FIG. 9.**

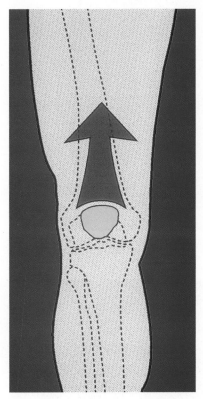

**FIG. 10.**

## TIPS

1. A simultaneous block of the femoral cutaneous, femoral, and obturator nerves, referred to as a 3-in-1 block, can be achieved by applying pressure with one hand immediately distal to the needle. The femoral, lateral femoral, femoral cutaneous, and obturator innervation is shown in **Fig. 11**. To avoid any changes in the needle position relative to the nerve, it is recommended to position the hand properly for performing a 3-in-1 block at the initial phase of the block rather than at the time of injection of the local anesthetic solution. The obturator and the femoral cutaneous nerves can be blocked individually **(Fig. 12)**.

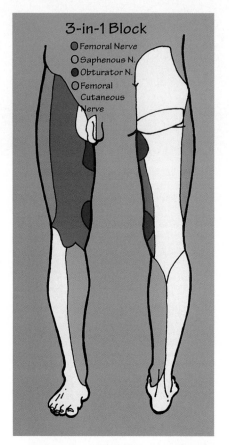

**FIG. 11.**

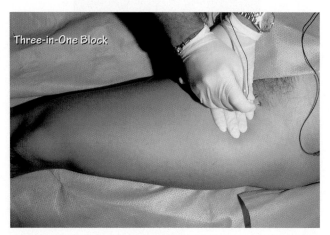

**FIG. 12.**

2.  To block the obturator nerve, half of a square with a side of 2 cm is drawn lateral to the pubic tubercle. A 100-mm b-beveled needle is introduced perpendicular to the skin. Within a short distance (~3 cm), the pubis bone is felt. The needle is redirected laterally into the obturator canal for another 2 cm. After negative blood aspiration, the local anesthetic solution is injected.

3.  To block the lateral femoral cutaneous nerve, half of a square with a side of 2 cm is drawn medial to the anterior superior iliac spine. At this point, a 22-gauge, 40-mm needle is introduced until a pop is felt (passage through the fascia lata). A volume of 10 to 15 ml of local anesthetic solution is sprayed around the area **(Fig. 13)**.

4.  If a tourniquet is not required or the obturator or lateral femoral cutaneous nerves do not need to be blocked, it is possible to block the femoral nerve after blocking the sciatic nerve when using an anterior approach, as previously described.

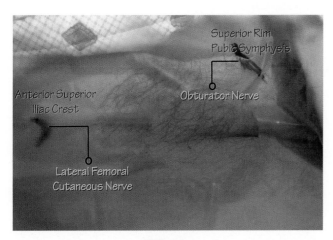

**FIG. 13.**

## SUGGESTED READINGS

Capellino A, Jokl P, Ruwe PA. Regional anesthesia in knee arthroscopy: a new technique involving femoral and sciatic nerve blocks in knee arthroscopy. *Arthroscopy* 1996;12:120–123.

Gjessing J, Harley N. Sciatic and femoral nerve block with mepivacaine for surgery on the lower limb. *Anaesthesia* 1969;24:213–218.

Jankowski CJ, Horlocker TT, Rock MJ, Stuart MJ. Femoral 3-in-1 nerve block decreases recovery room time and charges and time to hospital discharge after outpatient knee arthroscopy. *Reg Anesth and Pain Med* 1998;23S:60.

Parks CR, Kennedy WF. Obturator nerve block: a simplified approach. *Anesthesiology* 1967;28:775–778.

Winnie AP, Ramamurthy S, Durrani Z. The inguinal paravascular technique of lumbar plexus anesthesia: the 3-in-1 block. *Anesth Analg* 1973;52:989–996.

# 12

# Ankle Block

Gregory A. Liguori

**Patient Position:** Supine, with the leg free to rotate internally and externally.
**Needle Size:** 25-gauge, 50-mm.
**Volume:** 15 to 20 ml (15 ml can be used in each foot for bilateral blocks).
**Anatomic Landmarks:** There are five nerves supplying sensation to the foot **(Fig. 1)**; four are branches of the sciatic nerve (sural, posterior tibial, deep peroneal, and superficial peroneal) and one is a branch of the femoral nerve (saphenous).

• The posterior tibial nerve lies posterior and deep to the posterior tibial artery, approximately midway between the medial malleolus and the Achilles tendon. It is in a plane superficial to the tibia and deep to the flexor retinaculum. The posterior tibial nerve divides into the medial plantar nerve, the lateral plantar nerve and the calcaneal nerve.
• The deep peroneal nerve courses distally with the anterior tibial artery and, at the level of the malleoli, lies deep to the extensor retinaculum and superficial to the tibia. It is bounded medially by the tendon of the extensor hallucis longus and laterally by the anterior tibial artery.
• The superficial peroneal nerve travels distally with the peroneus brevis muscle and becomes superficial several centimeters proximal to the malleoli.
• The sural nerve courses superficially with the small saphenous vein and lies subcutaneously between the Achilles tendon and the lateral malleolus.

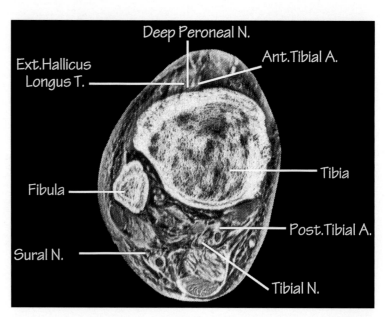

**FIG. 1.**

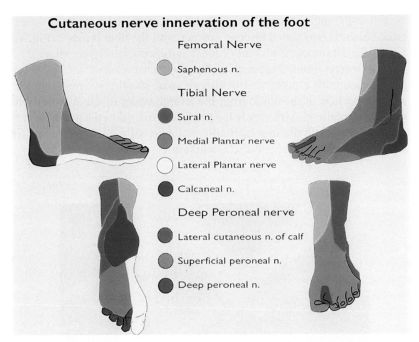

**Cutaneous nerve innervation of the foot**

Femoral Nerve

○ Saphenous n.

Tibial Nerve

● Sural n.

● Medial Plantar nerve

○ Lateral Plantar nerve

● Calcaneal n.

Deep Peroneal nerve

● Lateral cutaneous n. of calf

● Superficial peroneal n.

● Deep peroneal n.

**FIG. 2.**

- The saphenous nerve courses superficially with the great saphenous vein, where it divides into many small cutaneous branches. Innervation of the foot is shown in **Fig. 2**.

  **Approach and Technique:** The ankle block is performed using two needle punctures.

1. Block of the posterior tibial nerve: the leg is externally rotated with the knee flexed. The posterior tibial artery is palpated at the inferior border of the medial malleolus and 1 to 2 cm anterior to the Achilles tendon **(Fig. 3)**. The needle is directed posterior to the artery and advanced until the flexor retinaculum is pierced or bone contact with the tibia is made. Five to 10 ml of local anesthetic is injected after a negative aspiration.
2. Block of the deep and superficial peroneal, saphenous, and sural nerve.
   a. Block of the deep peroneal nerve is accomplished by asking the patient to extend the foot and first toe against resistance. This allows palpation of the extensor digitorum and extensor hallucis longus tendons above the ankle joint at the level of the malleoli. The needle is directed perpendicular to the skin,

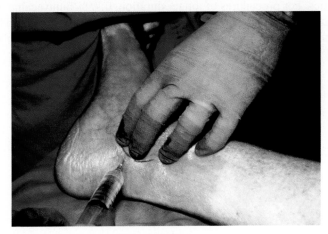

**FIG. 3.**

medial to the anterior tibial artery and between the tendons until the extensor retinaculum is penetrated or bone contact with the tibia is made **(Fig. 4)**. After a negative aspiration, 2 to 4 ml of local anesthetic solution is injected.

   b. The saphenous, sural, and superficial peroneal nerves and their distal branches are blocked with a subcutaneous ring of local anesthetic extending across the anterior portion of the ankle from the lateral aspect of the Achilles tendon to the medial malleoli. This ring is located just proximal to the malleoli. It is often necessary to rotate the foot internally and externally to complete this ring and inject 4 to 8 ml of local anesthetic solution.

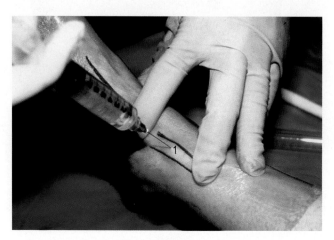

**FIG. 4.**

### TIPS

1. Infiltration of local anesthetic during an ankle block can be uncomfortable, especially during blockade of the superficial nerves. Therefore, it is important to provide the patient with appropriate sedation.

2. A pop is sometimes felt as the needle passes through the flexor retinaculum (posterior tibial) or extensor retinaculum (deep peroneal). This pop is often difficult to appreciate; therefore, the use of bone contact is more reliable. A diffuse fullness can often be noted on injection of local anesthetic around the deep nerves. If a paresthesia is noted, the needle is withdrawn and redirected slightly.

3. Two percent lidocaine or 1.5% mepivacaine are appropriate for procedures of short duration. However, little postoperative analgesia is provided (3 to 5 hours) with these anesthetics. For procedures of longer duration, 0.75% bupivacaine is very effective in producing long-acting anesthesia (6 to 8 hours) and analgesia (up to 24 hours). Although experience remains anecdotal, it seems that a combination of 0.75% bupivacaine and 2% lidocaine produces analgesia of intermediate duration.

4. The use of epinephrine in ankle blocks is contraindicated because the local anesthetic is injected perivascularly at both major arteries of the foot. Systemic absorption of local anesthetic from an ankle block is minimal; in addition, if a longer duration of action is desired, the choice of local anesthetic should be altered (i.e., bupivacaine in place of lidocaine), or a low dose of clonidine may be added to the block.

5. A variation of this technique that is highly effective is a midtarsal approach.

6. The addition of 10 μg/ml clonidine to lidocaine increases the duration and the quality of the block.

## SUGGESTED READINGS

Mineo R, Sharrock N. Venous levels of lidocaine and bupivacaine after midtarsal ankle block. *Reg Anesth* 1992;17:47–49.

Reinhart D, Wang W, Stagg K, et al. Post-operative analgesia after peripheral nerve block for podiatric surgery: clinical efficacy and chemical stability of lidocaine alone versus lidocaine plus clonidine. *Anesth Analg* 1996;83:760–765.

Sharrock N, Waller J, Fierro L. Midtarsal block for surgery of the forefoot. *Br J Anaesth* 1986; 58:37–40.

# 13

# Cervical Block

Pierre-Georges Durand, Vincent Piriou,
and Jean-Jacques Lehot

**Patient Position:** Supine, with head turned away from side where block is to be performed.

**Indications:** Carotid endarterectomy.

**Needle Size:** 22-gauge, 38-mm for deep cervical block (B. Braun/McGaw Medical, Inc., Bethlehem, PA); 22-gauge, 70-mm for superficial cervical block (B. Braun/McGaw Medical, Inc., Bethlehem, PA).

**Volume:** 30 to 45 ml.

**Anatomic Landmarks:** A line is drawn from 1 cm behind the tip of the mastoid process to the transverse process of the sixth cervical vertebrae (C6; identified by a vertical line drawn from the superior tip of the thyroid cartilage). On this line, C2 is 2 cm beneath the mastoid process, C3 is 1.5 cm beneath C2, and C4 is 1.5 cm beneath C3 **(Fig. 1).**

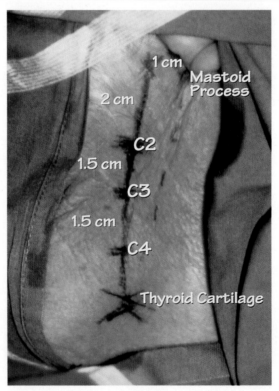

FIG. 1.

## APPROACH AND TECHNIQUE

### Deep Cervical Block

A needle is inserted medially as well as slightly caudally to obtain contact with the transverse processes of the C2, C3, and C4. The local anesthetic solution is slowly administered near the transverse process: 4 to 7 ml of 0.5% bupivacaine, or 6 to 10 ml of 0.25% bupivacaine, or 10 ml of a mixture of equal proportions of 0.25% bupivacaine and 1% lidocaine **(Fig. 2)**.

*Note:* The cervical block can also be performed with a single injection at the C3 or C4 level of 20 to 25 ml of local anesthetic solution (the solution diffuses into the paravertebral space).

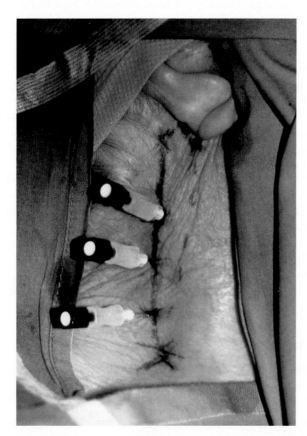

**FIG. 2.**

## Superficial Cervical Block

Twenty to 25 ml of 1% lidocaine is infiltrated into the deep subcutaneous from C3 anteriorly toward the mastoid process to a point 2 cm superior to the clavicle.

## TIPS

1. Cooperation of the patient is mandatory. Therefore, premedication and intraoperative sedation should be as light as possible. Benzodiazepines are not recommended because of the possible associated disorientation.
2. Immediate central nervous system (CNS) toxicity may occur from an intravascular or subarachnoid administration.
3. CNS toxicity occurring within 30 minutes of local anesthetic administration may be due to overdosage. The surgeon must administer 5 to 10 ml lidocaine next to the carotid bifurcation with an injection or a swab.
4. Paralysis of the phrenic nerve is possible: only one side is anesthetized on the same day, particularly in obese patients or those with chronic respiratory failure. Pulse oxygen saturation is mandatory.
5. An oxygen nasal catheter is more comfortable than a facial mask.
6. Other facial nerve paralysis are rare and transient. Glossopharyngeal nerve (IX)—deglutition trouble, hypersalivation, and anesthesia of the posterior part of the tongue; vagal nerve (X)—dysphonia; spinal nerve (XI)—paralysis of sternocleidomastoid muscle, dysphonia, and deglutition trouble; great hypoglossal nerve (XII)—deviation of the tongue.
7. During carotid clamping, motricity of the contralateral hand is monitored through a pressure-activated musical toy.
8. Blood pressure and electrocardiography with ST segment monitoring are recommended during and after anesthesia.
9. In atheromatous patients, head hyperextension or excessive rotation can lead to cerebral ischemia.
10. The addition of clonidine reduces the incidence of tachycardia, a complication that occurs in 60% of patients undergoing cervical plexus block with lidocaine and epinephrine.

## SUGGESTED READINGS

Corson JD, Chang BB, Shah DM, Leather RP, De Leo BM, Karmody AM. The influence of anesthetic choice on carotid endarterectomy outcome. *Arch Surg* 1987;122:807–812.

Molnar RR, Davies MJ, Scott DA, Silbert BS, Mooney PH. Comparison of clonidine and epinephrine in lidocaine for cervical plexus block. *Reg Anesth* 1997;22:137–142.

Tettenborn B, Caplan LR, Sloan MA, et al. Postoperative brainstem and cerebellar infarcts. *Neurology* 1993;43:471–477.

Tissot S, Frering B, Gagnieu MC, Vallon JJ, Motin J. Plasma concentrations of lidocaine and bupivacaine after cervical plexus block. *Anesth Analg* 1997;84:1377–1379.

Winnie AP, Ramamurthy S, Durrani Z, Radonjic R. Interscalene cervical plexus block: a single-injection technique. *Anesth Analg* 1975;54:370–375.

# 14

# Peribulbar Block

Didier Sciard

**Patient Position:** Supine, eyes closed in a central position.

**Indications:** Anterior eye segment surgery—cataract, trabeculectomy; posterior eye segment surgery—vitreoretinal surgery; conjunctival surgery, scleral buckle.

**Needle Size:** 23 gauge, 25 mm, normal bevel.

**Local Anesthetic Solution:** Half 0.5% or 0.75% bupivacaine, half 2% lidocaine, plus 100 to 150 UI/10 ml hyaluronidase.

**Volume:** 8 to 12 ml.

**Anatomic Landmarks:** Inferotemporal orbit injection—third inferolateral border of the orbit; superonasal orbit injection—third superomedial border of the orbit.

## APPROACH AND TECHNIQUES

### Inferotemporal Pericone Injection

The needle is introduced perpendicular to the skin. After contact with the bony rim, the needle is moved slightly in the cranial direction to lose this bone contact, angled 30 degrees, and introduced another 5 mm to a new periosteum contact. The needle is then moved back to the perpendicular position and progressively inserted to its full extent. After a negative blood aspiration, 6 to 8 ml of local anesthetic solution is injected. A good sign is a relative protrusion of the eye with a downward movement of the superior eyelid during the injection. Ocular tonicity must be checked continuously during the procedure **(Figs. 1, 2).**

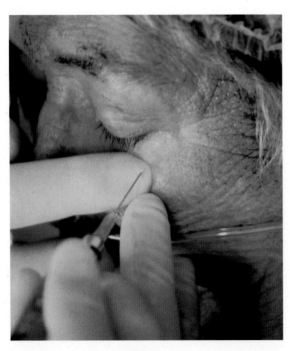

FIG. 1.

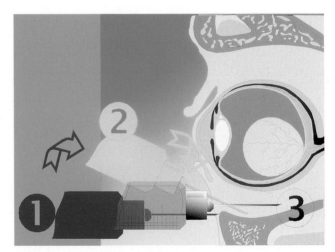

FIG. 2.

## Superonasal Pericone Injection

The technique is similar to the one described for the inferotemporal injection. The needle is moved slightly in the caudal direction, and 2 to 4 ml of local anesthetic solution is injected **(Figs. 3, 4)**.

*After these injections, the globe is compressed* for 5 to 10 minutes with a special device such as a Hoonan's balloon. The low-pressure cuff allows for ocular compression of less than 30 mm Hg **(Fig. 5)**.

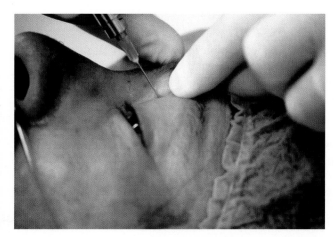

FIG. 3.

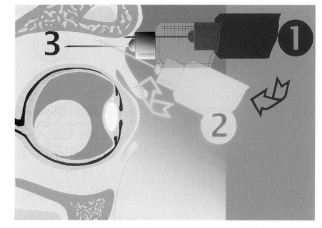

FIG. 4.

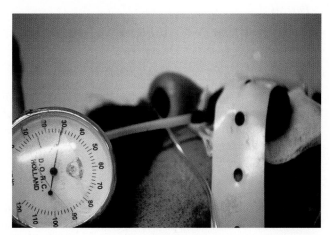

FIG. 5.

### Evaluation of the Block

The potency of the motor block is evaluated using the akinesia score: the patient is asked to open his or her eye (0 to 2), to look up (0 to 2), to look down (0 to 2), and to move laterally on one side (0 to 2) and on the other side (0 to 2). The total score varies from zero to 10. A block with a score of at least 8 is considered satisfactory. The quality of the sensory blockade can be verified by testing conjunctival sensitivity to touch or topical drugs.

### Complications

#### Ocular Perforation

There is an increased risk of ocular perforation in patients with large eyes (near-sighted). In addition, in patients with a small orbital cavity, the risk of ocular perforation is especially increased during the superonasal injection.

#### Retrobulbar Hemorrhage

The risk is increased in elderly patients treated with steroids or aspirin and other nonsteroidal anti-inflammatory drugs.

#### Infection

The risk of infection after peribulbar block is minimal because of the bacteriostatic property of the local anesthetic solution and the use of aseptic technique.

#### Paresis

There is a light risk of paresis of the upper eyelid with the superonasal approach.

#### Central Nervous System Side Effects

The risk of injection into the optic nerve sheath (resulting in unexpected intradural injection, requiring general anesthesia and tracheal intubation) or intravascular injection (producing centrally mediated cardiovascular or respiratory depression) is minimal with this approach.

### TIPS

1. This block allows for most types of intraocular surgery to be performed with a lower risk of neural optic damage or intradural or intravascular injection than the retrobulbar block. Use of the retrobulbar block should be reserved to ophthalmologists.

2. *Sedation*: The use of sedation before injection is indicated to decrease anxiety and minimize recall. During the procedure, the patient's cooperation is important, and therefore excessive use of sedative drugs is not advisable. However, in patients with major respiratory or neuromuscular diseases, sedation is contraindicated. In this instance, the use of topical anesthesia with a transconjunctival injection represents an alternative.

3. *Needle*: (a) The normal bevel increases the needle's penetration power (less painful) and does not increase the risk of ocular perforation. In addition, in case of perforation, the damage done to the globe is decreased. (b) The needle's length must be less than 30 mm to lower the risk of neural optic damage (unexpected retrobulbar injection).

4. *Drugs*: Mepivacaine 2% gives a good motor block and can be used alone instead of the mixture of lidocaine and bupivacaine. When a prolonged sensory block is

required (vitreoretinal surgery), 1 μg/kg clonidine can be added to the solution of local anesthetic. Ropivacaine 7.5% can also be used as a long-acting local anesthetic.

5. *Medial canthus (caruncula) approach*: This approach can be used to complement an incomplete peribulbar block. The puncture is done just above the caruncula, in the semilunaris fold. The needle is directed primarily to the nose and is inserted perpendicular to the eye with a constant pressure, producing a slight attraction of the eye. During the introduction of the needle, a loss of resistance is indicated by the eye returning to a central position. After a negative blood aspiration, 6 to 10 ml of the local anesthetic solution is injected. The caruncula approach can also be used as the sole approach for a peribulbar block. However, there is an increased risk of paresis of the medial rectus muscle, which is temporary most of the time but requires physical therapy in a few cases.

## SUGGESTED READINGS

Brydon CW, et al. An evaluation of two concentrations of hyaluronidase for supplementation of peribulbar anaesthesia. *Anaesthesia* 1995;50:998–1000.

Crawford M, et al. The effect of hyaluronidase on peribulbar block. *Anaesthesia* 1994;49:907–908.

Davis DB II, Mandel MR. Efficacy and complication rate of 16,224 consecutive peribulbar blocks: a prospective multicenter study. *J Cataract Refract Surg* 1994;20:327–337.

Dick B, Jacobi FK. Cataract surgery and anticoagulation current status. *Klin Monatsbl Augenheilkd* 1996;209:340–346.

Gomez RS, Andrade LOF, Rezende Costa JR. Brainstem anaesthesia after peribulbar anaesthesia. *Can J Anaesth* 1997;44:732–734.

Haimeur C, et al. Peribulbar anesthesia for cataract surgery. *Cah Anesthesiol* 1995;21:16–20.

Hamilton RC. Complications of retrobulbar and peribulbar blocks. *Reg Anesth* 1990;15:106–107.

Hamilton RC. Techniques of orbital regional anaesthesia. *Br J Anaesth* 1995;75:88–92.

McCombe M, Heriot W. Penetrating ocular injury following local anaesthesia. *Aust N Z J Ophthalmol* 1995;23:33–36.

Ripart J, Lefrant JY, Eledjam JJ. Medial canthus (caruncle) single injection periocular anesthesia. *Anesth Analg* 1996;83:1234–1238.

Rubin AP. Complications of local anaesthesia for ophthalmic surgery. *Br J Anaesth* 1995;75:93–96.

# 15

# Intercostal Block

Sukhijinder Dhother

**Patient Position:** Prone with arms hanging downward to rotate scapulae away from midline. Pillow under abdomen and head turned to the side.

**Indications:** Pain relief from upper abdominal and thoracotomy incisions. Pain relief from fractured ribs.

**Needle Size:** 22-gauge, 38-mm needle and a three-ring 10-ml syringe (BD & Co., Franklin Lakes, NY).

**Volume:** 0.25% bupivacaine with 1/200,000 epinephrine, 3 to 5 ml per rib (0.5% bupivacaine if muscle relaxation is also needed.)

**Anatomic Landmarks:** Draw a line connecting the posterior spinous processes of T6-L5. Next draw paramedian lines at the posterior angle of the ribs, just lateral to the paraspinous muscles. (Mark 7 cm from midline along the lower border of T12 and at 5 cm from midline along lower border of T6, and join these points.) Connect these two points and mark the lower border of each intervening rib where it crosses this line **(Fig. 1).**

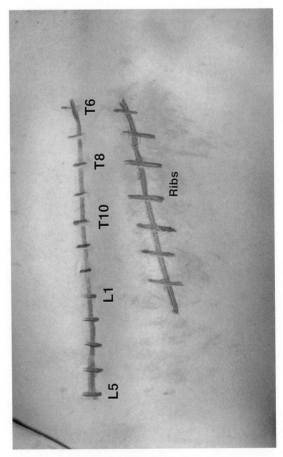

**FIG. 1.**

**Approach and Technique:** Using 1% lidocaine, create skin wheals at each marked injection site with 30-gauge needle **(Fig. 2)**. Standing at the side of the patient, begin at the lowest rib, using index and middle fingers of the cephalad hand to retract the wheal site up and over the rib. Insert block needle between tips of the retracting fingers until it just contacts the rib. Keep the needle steady and do not allow it to penetrate any deeper. Adjust cephalad hand so that the hub of the needle is now held between the thumb and index finger with the hypothenar eminence resting on the back. Keeping a 20-degree cephalad angle, walk the needle backward off the inferior margin of the rib. Now advance the depth by 2 to 4 mm past the edge of the rib into the intercostal groove. Inject 3 to 5 ml of anesthetic solution. Retract the needle. Reload the syringe, if necessary, and repeat for the next rib.

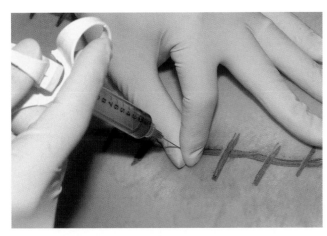

**FIG. 2.**

## TIPS

1. Adequate sedation needs to be provided to allow good tolerance of the procedure.
2. Practice hand and needle control.
3. Use the three-ring adapter for the syringe to allow better control during aspiration and injection.
4. There is a risk of pneumothorax (<1% in experienced hands).
5. It is important to confirm negative blood aspiration before any injection to prevent intravascular injection of local anesthetics.
6. To prevent systemic toxicity and complications of local anesthetic solutions, it is necessary to verify that the total dose is within the therapeutic range and to observe patient for the first 30 minutes after injections.

## SUGGESTED READINGS

Brown DL. *Atlas of regional anesthesia*. Philadelphia: WB Saunders, 1992.

Moore DC. Intercostal nerve block for postoperative somatic pain following surgery of thorax and upper abdomen. *Br J Anaesth* 1975;47:284–286.

Mulroy MF. *Regional anesthesia: an illustrated procedure guide*. Boston: Little, Brown & Company, 1989.

# 16
# Bier Block

Sukhijinder Dhother

**Patient Position:** Supine, with the extremity to be blocked supported on a side table extension.

**Indications:** Surgery of the arm below the level of the cuff, usually at or below the elbow. Duration not to exceed 90 minutes.

**Needle Size:** 20-gauge intravenous cannula in dorsum of hand and away from surgical site.

**Volume:** 1 ml/kg up to 60 ml 0.5% lidocaine.

**Anatomic Landmarks: A** convenient distal vein away from the surgical site; distal vein of the hand.

**Approach and Technique:** Insert and secure intravenous cannula **(Fig. 1).** Next, wrap upper arm with 10 cm Webril padding band (Kendall Healthcare, Mansfield, MA), then apply an appropriate sized pneumatic double cuff to the upper arm. The lower end of the distal cuff is secured with foam tape (10 cm) to prevent migration. Next, check the integrity of both cuffs by sequential inflation and deflation. The arm is elevated, and the patient is asked to close his hand firmly on a padding bandage **(Fig. 2).** A 10-cm latex bandage (Esmarch bandage, Rüsch, Inc., Duluth, GA) is wrapped from distal to proximal to provide exsanguination of the limb **(Fig. 3).** The proximal (upper) tourniquet is inflated to 100 mm Hg above systolic pressure, or at least 250 mm Hg, and then the latex bandage is removed. Absence of brachial and distal pulses indicates correct function. Fifty milliliters of 0.5% lidocaine is injected slowly. The cannula is removed and the arm prepared for surgery. Adequate sensory anesthesia should be achieved in approximately 10 to 15 minutes.

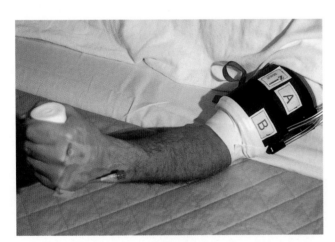

**FIG. 1.**

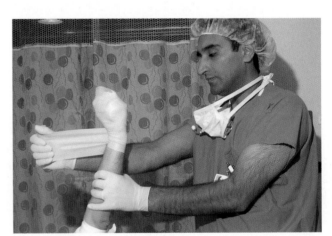

**FIG. 2.**

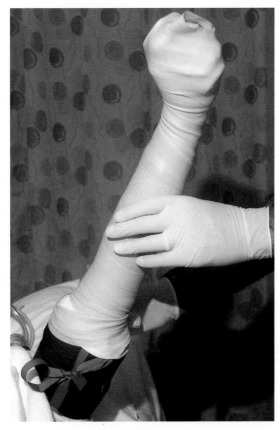

**FIG. 3.**

## TIPS

1. To prevent local anesthetic toxicity reactions, the tourniquet should remain in place for at least 45 minutes.
2. The patient should be asked to firmly close his or her hand around a tape role. This allows better exsanguination of the hand.
3. It is best to provide a tourniquet effect proximal to the patient's wrist by wrapping the operator's hand around it.
4. Inject half the anesthetic solution and observe the distension and backward filling of the veins. The remaining volume is then injected after releasing the wrist to allow a proximal spread up to the level of the proximal cuff.
5. When the patient begins experiencing tourniquet pain, it is time to inflate the distal cuff and deflate the proximal cuff, up to an additional 30 minutes. Do not deflate the cuffs until at least 20 minutes after injection. Be vigilant for signs of systemic absorption during tourniquet release.

## SUGGESTED READINGS

Brown DL. *Atlas of regional anesthesia*. Philadelphia: WB Saunders, 1992.
Holmes CM. Intravenous regional anesthesia: a useful method of producing analgesia of the limbs. *Lancet* 1963;1:245.
Mulroy MF. *Regional anesthesia: an illustrated procedural guide*. Boston: Little, Brown & Company, 1989.

# 17

# Airway Block

Carin A. Hagberg and Jacques E. Chelly

Innervation of the nasal, oropharyngeal, and laryngeal cavities, as well as the trachea, depends on three pairs of cranial nerves: the trigeminal (V), vagus (X), and glossopharyngeal (IX) nerves. Most of the nasal cavity innervation involves the sphenopalatine ganglion and the ethmoid nerve. Application of long cotton-tipped applicators soaked in 4% lidocaine with epinephrine or cocaine over the mucosa allows block of the sphenopalatine ganglion (applicator angled at 45 degrees to the hard palate) and the anterior ethmoid nerve (applicator parallel to the dorsal surface of the nose).

The glossopharyngeal nerve provides sensory innervation of the oropharynx, including the posterior third of the tongue, anterior surface of the epiglottis, posterior and lateral walls of the pharynx, and the tonsillar pillars. The glossopharyngeal nerve also provides motor innervation to the stylopharyngeus muscle, involved in deglutition. The rest of the pharynx, as well as the upper larynx, vocal cords, and trachea are innervated by the vagus nerve and its branches, especially the superior laryngeal and the recurrent laryngeal nerves.

Airway blocks usually benefit from administration of 0.4 to 0.8 mg intravenous glycopyrrolate (A.H. Robbins Co., Inc., Richmond, VA) to decrease the amount of secretions, and from the use of a vasoconstrictor for the nasal mucosa (1% phenylephrine [Sanofi Pharmaceuticals, Inc., New York NY]) in the absence of contraindications.

The following points need to be considered in the performance of airway blocks:

1. The risk-to-benefit ratio has to be established, taking into account (a) an alternative plan, including the direct spray of local anesthetic solution using 4% lidocaine or 14% to 20% benzocaine (risk of methemoglobinemia) or indirect spray with a nebulizer using 4% lidocaine; (b) the time available; and (c) the patient's condition, including level of consciousness and degree of respiratory depression or insufficiency.

2. It is important to maintain the patient comfortably by using appropriate sedation, usually a combination of 2 mg midazolam (Roche Laboratories, Nutley, NJ), 100 μg fentanyl, and 2.5 mg droperidol (SoloPak Pharmaceuticals, Inc., Boca Raton, FL). However, sedation should be individually titrated so that meaningful verbal contact with the patient is maintained.

Anesthesia practitioners often perform airway blocks in patients who require awake intubation. Practitioners should practice as much as possible in nonemergency situations to gain experience so that when a difficult intubation or emergency arises, the situation is handled appropriately.

## SUGGESTED READINGS

Bourke DL, Katz J, Tonneson A. Nebulized anesthesia for awake endotracheal intubation. *Anesthesiology* 1985;63:690–692.

Douglas WW, Fairbanks VF. Methemoglobinemia induced by a topical anesthetic spray (Cetacaine). *Chest* 1977;71:587–591.

Fry WA. Techniques of topical anesthesia for bronchoscopy. *Chest* 1978;73:694–696.

Gotta AW, Sullivan CA. Anaesthesia of the upper airway using topical anesthetic and superior laryngeal nerve block. *Br J Anaesth* 1981;53:1055–1058.

Kopman AF, Wollman SB, Ross K, et al. Awake endotracheal intubation: a review of 267 cases. *Anesth Analg* 1975;54:323–327.

O'Hollander AA, Monteny E, Dewachter B, Sanders M, Dubois-Primo J. Intubation under topical supra-glottic analgesia in unpremedicated and non-fasting patients: amnesic effects of sub-hypnotic doses of diazepam and Innovar. *Canadian Anaesthetists Society Journal* 1974;21:467–474.

Sidhu VS, Whitehead EM, Ainsworth QP, et al. A technique of awake fibreoptic intubation: experience in patients with cervical spine disease. *Anaesthesia* 1993;48:910–913.

# A. Glossopharyngeal Nerve Block

**Patient Position:** Supine.

**Indications:** Abolition of the gag reflex or hemodynamic response to laryngoscopy.

**Needle:** 25-gauge spinal needle.

**Local Anesthetic Solutions:** 2% lidocaine.

**Volume:** 2 to 4 ml per side.

**Anatomic Landmarks:** The glossopharyngeal nerve, which emerges from the skull through the jugular foramen and travels along the lateral wall of the pharynx.

**Approach and Technique:** The physician is situated on the contralateral side of the patient's head. With the patient's mouth wide open, a tongue blade is introduced into the mouth to displace the tongue laterally, creating a gutter between the tongue and the teeth. The gutter ends posteriorly in a cul-de-sac formed by the base of the palatoglossal arch. A 25-gauge spinal needle is inserted at the base of the cul-de-sac and advanced slightly (0.25 to 0.5 cm). Two milliliters of 2% lidocaine is injected after negative air and blood aspiration tests. The procedure is repeated on the other side **(Fig. 1).**

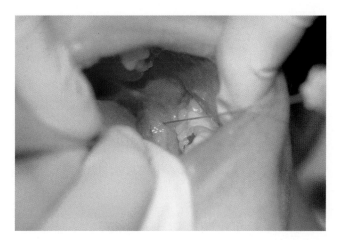

**FIG. 1.**

## TIPS

1. The use of a tongue blade may be facilitated by prior mouth topicalization with a local anesthetic solution. Also, 2% lidocaine jelly may be used, spread directly on the tongue blade.
2. If air is aspirated, the needle needs to be retrieved.
3. If blood is aspirated, the needle is redirected medially.

## SUGGESTED READINGS

Kazuhisa K, Norimasa S, Takanori M, et al. Glossopharyngeal nerve block for carotid sinus syndrome. *Anesth Analg* 1992;75:1036–1037.

Ovassapian A, Krejcie TC, Yelich SJ, et al. Awake fibreoptic intubation in the patient at high risk of aspiration. *Br J Anaesth* 1989;62:13–16.

Reed AF, Han DG. Preparation of the patient for awake intubation. *Anesthesiol Clin North Am* 1991; 9:69.

Rovenstein EA, Papper EM. Glossopharyngeal nerve block. *Am J Surg* 1948;75:713.

# B. Superior Laryngeal Nerve Block

**Patient Position:** Supine, head slightly extended.

**Indications:** Abolition of the gag reflex or hemodynamic response to laryngoscopy.

**Needle Size:** 23-gauge, 25-mm hypodermic needle.

**Local Anesthetic:** 2% lidocaine with epinephrine.

**Volume:** 2 to 4 ml.

**Anatomic Landmarks:** The superior laryngeal nerve supplies the sensory innervation of the larynx down to but excluding the vocal cords. At its origin, it travels with the vagus deep to the carotid artery, before becoming anterior. At the level of the cornu of the hyoid, it divides into an internal sensory branch and an external motor branch to the cricothyroid muscle. The internal branch pierces the thyrohyoid membrane along with the laryngeal artery and vein and splits into two branches. The ascending branch supplies the epiglottis and the vestibules of the larynx, whereas the descending branch supplies innervation to the mucosa at the level of the vocal cords.

**Approach and Technique:** The physician is situated on the ipsilateral side of the neck. The cornu of the hyoid bone is palpated transversally with the thumb and index finger on the side of the neck immediately beneath the angle of the mandible and anterior to the carotid artery. To facilitate its identification, the hyoid bone is displaced toward the side being blocked **(Fig. 2).** One hand displaces the carotid artery laterally and posteriorly. With the other hand, a 25-mm, 23-gauge needle is walked off the cornu of the hyoid bone in an anterocaudal direction, aiming in the direction of the thyroid ligament. At a depth of 1 to 2 cm, a volume of 2 ml of 2% lidocaine with epinephrine is injected after negative air and blood aspiration **(Fig. 3).**

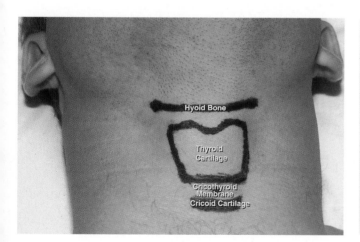

FIG. 2.

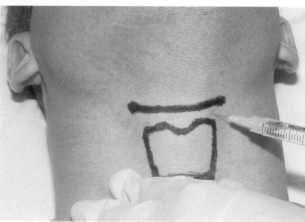

FIG. 3.

**TIPS**

1. If air is aspirated, the laryngeal mucosa has been pierced and the needle needs to be retrieved.
2. If blood is aspirated (superior artery or vein), the needle need to be redirected anteriorly. Pressure is applied to avoid hematoma formation.
3. If laryngeal evaluation is performed for vocal cord movement, only the internal laryngeal nerve needs to be blocked. For this purpose, the patient is asked to open his or her mouth widely. The tongue is depressed with a tongue blade and pulled laterally. A Krause forceps armed with cotton soaked with 4% lidocaine is placed over the lateral posterior curvature of the tongue until resistance is met. The forceps should remain in this position for 5 minutes, and the procedure is then repeated on the opposite side.
4. In case of bronchoscopy or awake intubation, the superior laryngeal and the recurrent laryngeal nerves need to be blocked.

## SUGGESTED READINGS

Benumof JL. Management of the difficult airway. *Anesthesiology* 1991;75:1087–1110.

Gotta AW, Sullivan CA. Superior laryngeal nerve block: an aid to intubating the patient with fractured mandible. *J Trauma* 1984;24:83–85.

Hunt LA, Boyd GL. Superior laryngeal nerve block as a supplement to total intravenous anesthesia for rigid laser bronchoscopy in a patient with myasthenic syndrome. *Anesth Analg* 1992;75:458–460.

Reed AF, Han DG. Preparation of the patient for awake intubation. *Anesthesiol Clin North Am* 1991;9:69.

Reed AP. Preparation of the patient for awake flexible fiberoptic bronchoscopy. *Chest* 1992;101:244–253.

Sidhu VS, Whitehead EM, Ainsworth QP, et al. A technique of awake fibreoptic intubation: experience in patients with cervical spine disease. *Anaesthesia* 1993;48:910–913.

# C. Recurrent Laryngeal Nerve Block

**Patient Position:** Supine with the neck hyperextended.

**Indications:** Laryngoscopy of the airway, awake intubation, and evaluation of vocal cord movements.

**Needle Size:** 21-gauge, 2.5-cm hypodermic needle.

**Volume:** 2% lidocaine, 3 to 4 ml.

**Anatomic Landmarks:** The right recurrent laryngeal nerve originates at the level of the right subclavian artery and loops around the innominate artery on the right and the aortic arch on the left. This nerve supplies sensory innervation to the vocal cords and the trachea, as well as motor innervation to the vocal cords.

**Approach and Technique:** With the physician standing so that his or her nondominant side faces the patient, the cricothyroid membrane is located and a small amount of local anesthesia is administered subcutaneously using a tuberculin syringe filled with 1% lidocaine. The nondominant hand is used to identify the cricothyroid membrane and to hold the trachea in place. A 10-ml syringe containing 2% lidocaine mounted on a 23-gauge needle is introduced into the trachea through the cricothyroid membrane at an angle of 45 degrees in a caudal direction. Immediately after its introduction into the trachea, a loss of resistance and the ability to aspirate air should occur. The patient is then asked to take a deep breath. At the end of the inspiratory effort, 3 to 4 ml of local anesthetic solution is injected into the trachea. The needle is removed, and the patient is asked to cough to distribute the anesthetic solution in the trachea and into the vocal cords **(Fig. 4).**

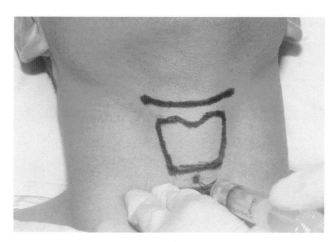

**FIG. 4.**

## TIPS

1. Before any maneuver, the patient needs to be informed that the injection of local anesthetic solution will likely make the him or her cough.
2. During performance of the block, the patient should not talk, swallow, or cough, if possible.
3. This block is contraindicated in patients diagnosed with an unstable neck.

## SUGGESTED READINGS

Benumof JL. Management of the difficult airway. *Anesthesiology* 1991;75:1087–1110.
Bonica JJ. Transtracheal anesthesia for endotracheal intubation. *Anesthesiology* 1949;10:736.
Gold MI, Buechael DR. Translaryngeal anesthesia: a review. *Anesthesiology* 1959;20:181.
Reed AP. Preparation of the patient for awake flexible fiberoptic bronchoscopy. *Chest* 1992;101:244–253.

# 18

# Thoracic Paravertebral Block

Jerry D. Vloka and Admir Hadžić

**Patient Position:** Sitting, with neck flexed.

**Common Indications:** Surgery (e.g., total mastectomy or axillary dissection); pain management (e.g., cholecystectomy, thoracotomy).

**Needle:** 22-gauge, 90-mm spinal needle (Quincke type).

**Volume:** 5 to 6 ml per level.

**Anatomic Landmarks:** The paravertebral space is limited anteriorly by the parietal pleura, posteriorly by the superior costotransverse ligament, and medially by the posterolateral aspect of the vertebra and the intervertebral foramen. The spinous process is the main landmark for this block.

**Approach and Technique:** The patient is in the sitting position with the neck flexed, so that the chin touches the chest. The spinal processes are palpated and marked with a skin marker **(Fig. 1)**. The insertion points are marked 2.5 cm lateral to the superior border of the spinal process, and infiltrated with local anesthetic. A 22-

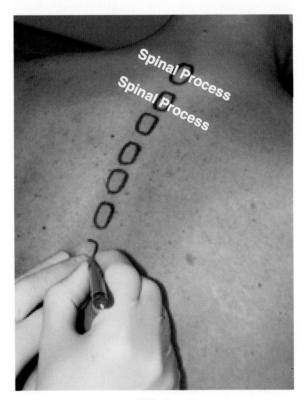

**FIG. 1.**

gauge, 90-mm spinal needle attached to tubing and syringe with local anesthetic is inserted perpendicular to the skin and advanced 2 to 4 cm until the transverse process of the respective vertebra is contacted. The needle is then withdrawn to the skin and reinserted to walk off the superior aspect of the transverse process. The needle is advanced 1 to 1.5 cm past the premeasured skin-to-bone distance. After negative aspiration, 5 to 6 ml of local anesthetic is injected at each level to be blocked **(Fig. 2)**.

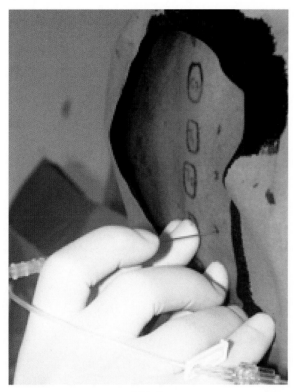

**FIG. 2.**

## TIPS

1. A total mastectomy requires a blockade extending from the C7 to T6 level.
2. A fast onset and most consistent results for surgical anesthesia are achieved with a mixture with equal volumes of 1.5% alkalinized mepivacaine (1 mEq of $NaHCO_3$/30 ml of mepivacaine) with 1:200,000 epinephrine and 0.5% bupivacaine.
3. Resistance on injection of local anesthetic is likely due to the needle tip being positioned in the superior costotransverse ligament. In this case, the needle should simply be advanced 1 to 2 mm.

## SUGGESTED READINGS

Coveney E, Weltz CR, Greengrass R, et al. Use of paravertebral block anesthesia in the surgical management of breast cancer. *Ann Surg* 1998;227:496–501.
Richardson J, Sabanathan S. Thoracic paravertebral analgesia. *Acta Anaesthesiol Scand* 1995;39: 1005–1015.

# SECTION III
# Continuous Peripheral Blocks

# 19

# General Concepts

F. Kayser Enneking

# A. Catheter Placement for Continuous Regional Anesthesia

Catheter placement to extend regional anesthesia has become a popular technique as improved outcome has been tied to improved postoperative analgesia. The next chapters describe the step-by-step placement of various catheters, but there are some general guidelines for catheter placement that may be helpful.

1. Orient the bevel of the introducing needle along the same axis as the nerve. Then, approach the nerve at the least acute angle as possible.

2. With the needle ideally placed, inject a mass of local anesthetic or normal saline to open up the fascial compartment. If the catheter is not threading easily after passing the tip of the needle, place the adapter on the end of the catheter and inject 3 ml of fluid through the catheter to open up the space, then try to advance the catheter again.

3. Introduce the catheter firmly, but if it does not thread, do not force it and kink it. Instead, try to lower the angle of the introducing needle, or change the orientation of the bevel of the introducing needle.

4. After the catheter has been successfully threaded, secure it! I remove the prep solution with sterile saline, swab the area with a clear adhesive, and then cover the catheter with a clear occlusive dressing.

5. Make sure to inject additional fluid. I prefer local anesthetic solution through the catheter after it is placed to ensure its potency. It is much easier to adjust it when you first put it in than later.

6. The patient should be given a bolus of local anesthetic to initiate the block, then started on a continuous infusion. The most common infusion solutions used for continuous regional analgesia are 0.25% to 0.125% bupivacaine or 0.2% ropivacaine. These solutions are then infused at a rate of 4 to 12 ml/hr depending on how the wound is drained, the size of the patient, and the intensity of pain experienced by the patient.

# B. Local Anesthetic Solution for Continuous Infusion

1. Local anesthetic is the primary component of peripheral nerve block infusion solutions. Bupivacaine, lidocaine, and ropivacaine are the most commonly used agents. Of these, bupivacaine has been the most commonly used for continuous peripheral nerve blocks. Typically, it is used as a 0.25% solution and run at a rate of 0.25 mg/kg/hr. At this concentration, motor block may occur. Ropivacaine, in a 0.2% solution run at a rate of 0.3 to 0.4 mg/kg/hr, may provide a better alternative to bupivacaine. During continuous epidural infusions of 0.1%, 0.2%, and 0.3% ropivacaine solutions or 0.25% bupivacaine, there was less motor block in all ropivacaine groups compared with the bupivacaine group. This separation of motor and sensory blockade may result in improved participation in active rehabilitation.

2. Unlike epidural infusions, and although there is a sound theoretic basis, the addition of narcotics to peripheral nerve blocks does not consistently enhance analgesia. To date, there has been no data published that support the addition of narcotics to continuous infusion solutions.

3. Clonidine (Boehringer Ingelheim Pharmaceuticals, Inc., Ridgefield, CT) may have a role in continuous peripheral nerve block infusions. In single-injection peripheral nerve blocks, it prolongs analgesia by 50% to 100%. In continuous infusions combined with dilute local anesthetics, clonidine at 1 µg/ml provides profound analgesia after ankle surgery. In the small doses recommended, clonidine does not appear to have any side effects.

4. Patients do not require extensive monitoring during continuous peripheral nerve blockade. If the extremity remains anesthetic, care must be taken to ensure it is protected and appropriately padded. The most important safety aspects are using a device that does not allow for inadvertent overdose and ensuring the proper dosage prescription. The most common symptoms of local anesthetic toxicity during continuous local anesthetic infusion are mental status changes, including sedation. Adding a patient-controlled mode of local anesthetic delivery may increase the safety of the technique by reducing the total dose of local anesthetic required for analgesia and high patient satisfaction.

## SUGGESTED READINGS

Borgeat A, Schappi B, Biasca N, Gerber C. Patient-controlled analgesia after major shoulder surgery. *Anesthesiology* 1997;87:1343–1347.

Eisenach JC, De Koch M, Klimischa W. Alpha(2) adrenergic agonists for regional anesthesia: a clinical review of clonidine (1984–1995). *Anesthesiology* 1996;85:655–674.

Emanuelsson BM, Zaric D, Nydahl PA, Axelsson KH. Pharmacokinetics of ropivacaine and bupivacaine during 21 hrs of continuous epidural infusion in healthy male volunteers. *Anesth Analg* 1995;81:1163–1168.

Enneking FK, Scarborough MT, Radson EA. Local anesthetic infusion through nerve sheath catheters for analgesia following upper extremity amputation: clinical report. *Reg Anesth* 1997; 22:351–356.

Singelyn FJ, Aye F, Gouverneur JM. Continuous popliteal sciatic nerve block: an original technique to provide postoperative analgesia after foot surgery. *Anesth Analg* 1997;84:383–386.

Singelyn FJ, Van der Elst P. Continuous 3-in-1 block after total hip replacement: continuous or patient-controlled infusion. *Anesth Analg* 1998;86[Suppl].

# 20

# Continuous Interscalene Block

Terese T. Horlocker

**Patient Position:** Supine, with head slightly turned to opposite side.

**Indications:** Shoulder surgery, including arthroscopic procedures. Continuous interscalene infusions are typically used to allow aggressive postoperative physical therapy and to maintain joint range of motion.

**Needle Size:** 18-gauge, 44.5-mm catheter over 20-gauge short-bevel introducer needle, and a 20-gauge catheter (Contiplex Continuous Nerve Block Set, B. Braun/McGaw Medical, Inc., Bethlehem, PA).

**Volume:** 20 ml followed by continuous infusion at the rate of 8 to 14 ml/hr starting within 1 hour of loading. A patient-controlled analgesic technique for continuous interscalene block has recently been described.

**Anatomic Landmarks:** Sternocleidomastoid muscle and interscalene groove. The patient is positioned supine with the head turned to the contralateral side. The interscalene groove is located by rolling the index finger laterally across the belly of the anterior scalene muscle to determine the groove between the anterior and middle scalene muscles. The needle insertion site is high in the interscalene groove, at the level of the sixth cervical vertebrae.

**Approach and Technique:** The modified perivascular technique allows easy catheter advancement because the needle approach is parallel to the brachial plexus sheath. However, the clinician must be able to visualize the nerves of the brachial plexus as they travel from the cervical foramen, through the interscalene groove, posteriorly to the midpoint of the clavicle, where they form terminal nerves at the level of the axilla. The needle is inserted *high* in the interscalene groove and advanced parallel to the long axis of the body. A paresthesia or nerve stimulator response usually occurs at a depth of approximately 2.5 cm **(Fig. 1)**. The catheter is advanced 5 cm into the sheath and secured. If the brachial plexus is not identified, the needle should be redirected laterally in small steps.

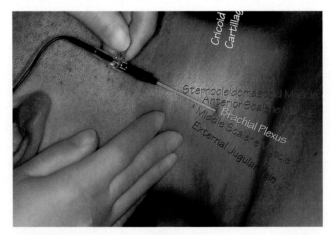

**FIG. 1.**

## TIPS

1. A marked rotation of the patient's head results in distortion of the anatomic landmarks and relationships.

2. Continuous interscalene block is best suited for shoulder surgery. High volumes of local anesthetic are required reliably to block the elbow, forearm, or hand.

3. Accurate identification of the interscalene groove is essential to both single-injection and continuous interscalene techniques. Do not be confused by the groove between the sternocleidomastoid and anterior scalene muscles! If the correct groove has been identified, the pulsation of the subclavian artery may be palpated.

4. Continuous catheter techniques often use large-gauge, blunt needles. Generous subcutaneous infiltration of local anesthetic increases patient comfort.

5. A shallow angle of needle insertion, with an approach parallel to the brachial plexus sheath, facilitates catheter placement.

6. An alternate classic approach to the perivascular technique uses a needle insertion angle and site identical to those with the single-dose interscalene block. (The needle is directed perpendicular to the skin, with a slightly caudal and posterior angulation.) However, catheter advancement may be difficult because the needle approaches the brachial plexus at a right angle, forcing the catheter to turn 90 degrees. Proximal advancement may result in cannulation of the epidural or intrathecal spaces.

7. The brachial plexus is near significant vascular and neural structures at the interscalene level. Meticulous regional technique must be used to avoid subarachnoid, epidural, and intravascular injection and cannulation.

8. Although there is a possibility of pneumothorax with the perivascular approach, this complication may be avoided by limiting the depth of needle insertion.

9. Phrenic nerve paralysis should be expected in all patients with a continuous interscalene infusion. Concentrations as low as 0.125% bupivacaine still result in a significant decrease in diaphragmatic motion and ventilatory function, which persists for the duration of the block.

10. This technique should not be used in patients who are unable to tolerate a 25% reduction in pulmonary function.

11. The high mobility of the cervical spine makes catheter dislodgment a common complaint. The perivascular approach allows catheter advancement of 5 to 10 cm, whereas only 2 to 3 cm may be possible with the classic approach. The improved catheter placement with the perivascular technique makes it the superior approach.

12. The stiff tip of the indwelling catheter combined with cervical and upper extremity movement may result in plexus irritation. Patients should be observed for new (nonsurgical) pain or neurologic complaints.

## SUGGESTED READINGS

Borgeat A, Schappi B, Biasca N, Gerber C. Patient-controlled analgesia after major shoulder surgery. *Anesthesiology* 1997;87:1343–1347.

Brown DL. Interscalene block. In: Brown DL, ed. *Atlas of regional anesthesia.* Philadelphia: WB Saunders, 1992:23–30.

DeKrey JA, Schroeder CF, Buechel DR. Continuous brachial plexus block. *Anesthesiology* 1969;30:332.

Pere P. The effect of continuous interscalene brachial plexus block with 0.125% bupivacaine plus fentanyl on diaphragmatic motility and ventilatory function. *Reg Anesth* 1993;18:93–97.

Ribeiro FC, Georgousis H, Bertram R, Scheiber G. Plexus irritation caused by interscalene brachial plexus catheter for shoulder surgery. *Anesth Analg* 1996;82:870–872.

Tuominen M, Haasio J, Hekali R, Rosenberg PH. Continuous interscalene brachial plexus block: clinical efficacy, technical problems and bupivacaine plasma concentrations. *Acta Anaesthesiol Scand* 1989;33:84–88.

Winnie AP, Collins VJ. The subclavian perivascular technique of brachial plexus anesthesia. *Anesthesiology* 1964;25:353–363.

# 21

# Continuous Infraclavicular Block

F. Kayser Enneking

**Patient Position:** Supine with the arm abducted 90 degrees at the shoulder. Preparation of the patient should include the anterior chest wall around the midpoint of the clavicle into the axilla.

**Indications:** Surgical anesthesia of the arm. Postoperative analgesia, particularly if early physical therapy is indicated.

**Needle Size:** 18-gauge, 150-mm insulated Tuohy needle and 20-gauge epidural catheter (Contiplex Insulated Tuohy Needle Set, B. Braun/McGaw Medical, Inc., Bethlehem, PA).

**Volume:** 40 ml initially, followed by 6 to 10 ml/hr.

**Anatomic Landmarks:** Axillary artery in the midportion of the axilla. This should be marked to give a visual clue to needle direction, 2.5 cm caudal to the midpoint of the clavicle for needle entry **(Fig. 1).**

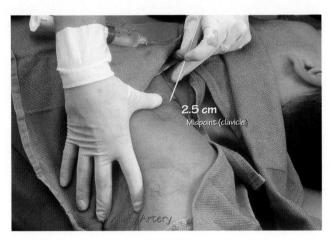

**FIG. 1.**

**Approach and Technique:** The operator stands on the side opposite the arm to be blocked. With one hand in the axilla, the other hand introduces the needle at the midpoint of the clavicle. The needle is directed laterally toward the axillary artery in the midportion of the axilla. This gives a rather flat trajectory to the needle. The first stimulation is of the pectoralis major muscle. Then, as the needle enters the axilla, the elements of the brachial plexus are stimulated **(Fig. 2)**; 20–40 cc of local anesthetic is injected. The catheter is then threaded 3 to 4 cms and secured on the anterior chest wall **(Figs. 3, 4)**.

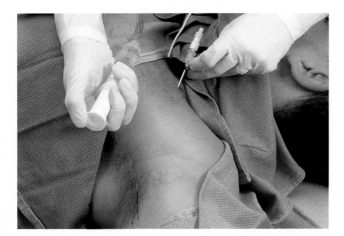

FIG. 2.

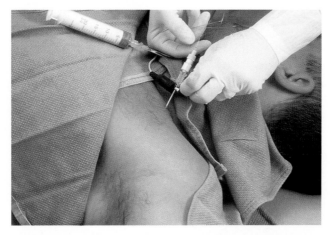

FIG. 3.

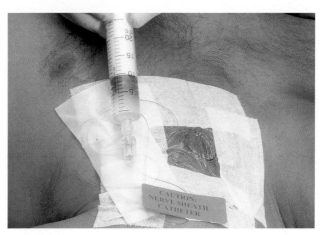

FIG. 4.

## TIPS

1. *Do not* overthread the catheter. The strong pectoralis muscle keeps the catheter firmly in place. If the catheter is threaded more than 4 cms, it may provide analgesia to a single nerve rather than the entire plexus.
2. By leaving his or her nondominant hand in the axilla, the operator can feel the needle enter the axilla even in a large patient.
3. To identify easily the needle entry site, the operator pretends he or she is inserting a subclavian line, but instead of going medially, goes laterally.

## SUGGESTED READING

Fitzgibbon DR, Debs AD, Erjavec MK. Selective musculocutaneous nerve block and infraclavicular brachial plexus anesthesia: case report. *Reg Anesth* 1995;20:239–241.

Steele SM, Klein SM, D'Ercole FJ, Greengrass RA, Gleason D. A new continuous catheter delivery system. *Anesth Analg* 1998;86:228–229.

# 22

# Continuous Axillary Block

F. Kayser Enneking

**Patient Position:** Arm abducted 90 degrees at the shoulder.

**Indications:** Surgical anesthesia from the elbow to the fingers. Postoperative pain relief and continuous sympathectomy.

**Needle Size:** 20-gauge pediatric Crawford epidural needle (Preferred Medical Products, Throrold, Ontario, Canada) or 18-gauge, 50-mm insulated Tuohy needle and 20-gauge epidural catheter (Contiplex Insulated Tuohy Needle Set, B. Braun/McGaw Medical, Inc., Bethlehem, PA).

**Volume:** 30 ml initially, with infusion of 6 to 10 ml/hr.

**Anatomic Landmarks:** Axillary artery into the lower portion of the axilla.

**Approach and Technique:** Palpation or Doppler signal identifies the axillary pulse. A skin nick is made with a sharp 18-gauge needle. The fingers are placed perpendicular along the course of the artery to stretch the skin tautly to allow the needle to be easily introduced **(Fig. 1)**. The stimulating needle is placed below the artery if a radial nerve block is specifically indicated, but above for all other procedures. The appropriate twitch is observed and the initial volume of local anesthetic is delivered. The catheter is introduced and threaded at least 5 cm **(Fig. 2)**.

If a nonstimulating technique is done, it is carried out with a blunt-tipped, short epidural catheter. The needle is introduced until a distinct pop is appreciated, the local anesthetic is injected, and then the catheter is threaded as described previously.

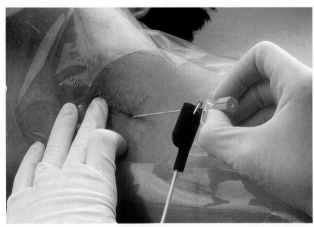

**FIG. 1.**

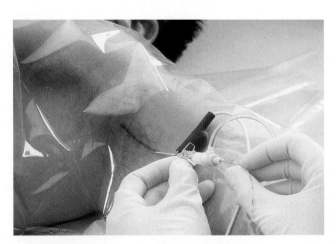

**FIG. 2.**

## TIPS

1. If the initial injection of local anesthetic is difficult, back the needle up by 1 mm, restimulate, and try to inject again. Difficulty with injection may indicate the needle is against a firm structure—not a nerve, it is hoped.
2. If the catheter does not thread, try the following:
   a. Inject 3 ml of local anesthetic through the catheter.
   b. Turn the bevel of the needle by 90 degrees.
   c. Withdraw the needle and catheter by 1 mm.
   d. If these do not work, you probably have located the nerve tangentially or you are still outside the sheath. Options then are to convert to a single-injection technique with a long-acting local anesthetic, or to start over.
3. Secure the catheter with benzoin, Steristrips, and a clear dressing. These catheters are notorious for working themselves out.

## SUGGESTED READINGS

Mezzatesta JP, Scott DA, Schweitzer SA, Selander DE. Continuous axillary brachial plexus block for postoperative pain relief: intermittent bolus versus continuos infusion. *Reg Anesth* 1997;22: 357–362.

Wajima Z, Shitara T, Kim C, et al. Comparison of continuous brachial plexus infusion of butorphanol, mepivacaine, and mepivacaine-butorphanol mixtures for postoperative analgesia. *Br J Anaesth* 1995;75:548–551.

# 23

# Continuous Blocks
# at the Wrist

Pascal Leclerc, Bernard Komly,
Thierry Garnier, Luc Mercadal, and
Bertrand Morel

**Patient Position:** The patient is in a supine position, with the arm placed with the palm facing upward.

**Indications:** Postoperative analgesia for early active physical therapy after finger and wrist surgery.

**Needle Size:** 18-gauge, 44.5-mm catheter over a 20-gauge short-bevel introducer needle and a 20-gauge catheter (Contiplex Continuous Nerve Block Set, B. Braun/McGaw Medical, Inc., Bethlehem, PA) for the median and ulnar nerves, and a 20-gauge epidural catheter (multiple holes at the tip) for the radial nerve.

**Volume:** Each nerve receives 6 to 8 ml of ropivacaine 0.2% plus clonidine 0.5 µg/kg every 12 hours for 3 to 5 days.

## ANATOMIC LANDMARKS

5 cm above the wrist crease.

### Ulnar Nerve

The ulnar nerve lies medial to the ulnar artery and under the flexor carpi ulnaris tendon, with the ulnar bone posterior.

### Median Nerve

The median nerve is located lateral to the palmaris longus tendon and medial to the flexor carpi radialis tendon.

### Radial Nerve

The radial nerve becomes subcutaneous 5 cm above the anatomic snuffbox.

## APPROACH AND TECHNIQUE

### Ulnar Nerve

A lateral approach to the flexor carpi ulnaris is preferred. The Contiplex catheter, connected to a nerve stimulator (B. Braun/McGaw Medical, Inc., Bethlehem, PA) set at 1.5 mA, is introduced below the flexor carpi ulnaris tendon and at a 45-degree angle, 5 to 7 cm above the wrist in the direction of the elbow **(Fig. 1)**. After an appropriate motor response (adduction of the thumb and metacarpophalangeal flexion of the long fingers) with a current of 0.6 mA, 6 to 8 ml of local anesthetic solution is injected. The catheter is introduced after removing the needle introducer **(Figs. 2, 3)**.

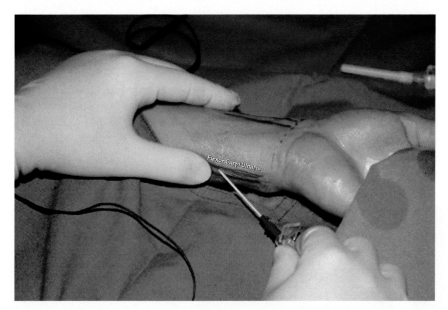

FIG. 1.

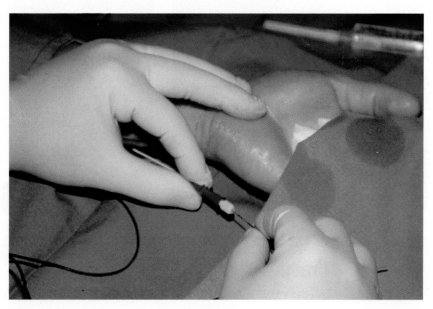

FIG. 2.

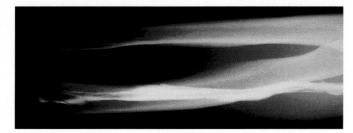

FIG. 3.

## Median Nerve

The 18-gauge Contiplex catheter with its introducer connected to a nerve stimulator set to deliver a current of 1.5 mA is introduced 4 to 5 cm above the wrist crease between the flexor carpi radialis and palmaris longus tendons at a 15- to 30-degree angle in the direction of the elbow **(Figs. 4, 5)**. After an appropriate motor response (opposition of the thumb by contraction of the thenar muscles, especially the opponens pollicis and abductor pollicis brevis) with a current of 0.6 mA, 6 to 8 ml of local anesthetic solution is injected. The catheter is introduced after removing the needle introducer **(Fig. 6)**.

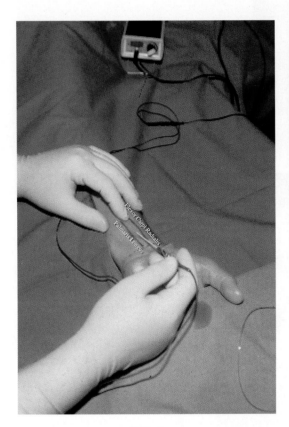

FIG. 4.

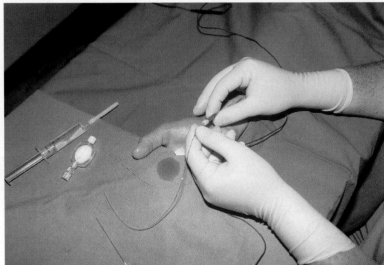

FIG. 5.

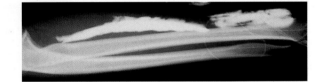

FIG. 6.

## Radial Nerve

The Contiplex catheter connected to a nerve stimulator set at 2 mA/200 msec (Stimuplex HNS11, B. Braun/McGaw Medical, Inc.) is introduced subcutaneously transversally over 3 cm, 5 cm above the styloid, to elicit paresthesia on the dorsal aspect of the hand **(Figs. 7, 8)**. Five to 8 ml of local anesthetic solution is infiltrated subcutaneously. After removing the needle introducer, an epidural catheter is introduced. The catheters are cut to the appropriate length and connected to a bacterial filter. They are kept in place with transparent tape (3M Health Care, St. Paul, MN) **(Fig. 9)**.

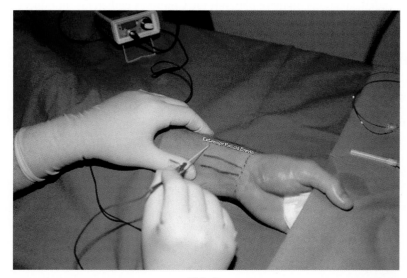

**FIG. 7.**

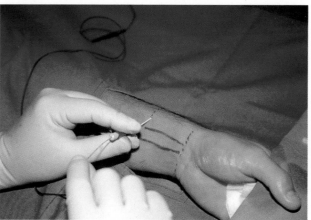

**FIG. 8.**

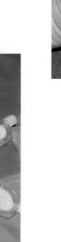

**FIG. 9.**

## TIPS

1. These blocks preserve motor function of the fingers (flexion and extension).
2. The use of a nerve stimulator is helpful for both the motor (ulnar and median) and sensory nerves (radial).
3. *Ulnar nerve:* The use of a lateral approach minimizes the risk of puncturing the ulnar artery.
4. *Median nerve:* Having the patient flex his or her wrist against resistance facilitates identification of the flexor carpi radialis tendon. Opposing the thumb and the little finger facilitates identification of the palmaris longus tendon.
5. *Median nerve:* 10% to 20% of patients have a fusion of their palmaris longus and flexor carpi radialis tendons. In these patients, the Contiplex catheter is introduced medial to the tendon and the median nerve is found under the tendon.

## SUGGESTED READINGS

Abrams R, Brown R, Botte M. The superficial branch of the radial nerve: an anatomic study with surgical implications. *J Hand Surg [Am]* 1993;17:1037–1041.

Kahle W, Leonhardt H, Platzer W. *Anatomie: système nerveux et organes des sens.* Vol 3. Paris: Flammarion, 1979:64–73.

Netter FH. *Atlas of human anatomy.* (Fr) Paris ed. Maloine-Plates 418–455, 1997.

# 24

# Continuous Sciatic Blocks

# A. Parasacral Approach

## Gary F. Morris and Jacques E. Chelly

**Patient Position:** The patient is positioned laterally with the operative limb uppermost. The hip and knee are slightly flexed to facilitate patient comfort.

**Indications:** Unilateral lower extremity surgery requiring prolonged postoperative pain control.

**Needle size:** 18-gauge, 150-mm insulated Tuohy needle and 20-gauge epidural catheter (Contiplex Insulated Tuohy Needle Set, B. Braun/McGaw, Bethlehem, PA).

**Volume:** 30 ml followed by 8 ml/hr infusion.

**Anatomic Landmarks:** The sacral plexus consists of nerve fibers originating from the L4-S3 nerve roots. These nerve roots travel within the pelvis anterior to the ischial bone and the piriformis muscle. They then coalesce to form the common peroneal, tibial, posterior femoral cutaneous, inferior gluteal, and superior gluteal nerves just before exiting the pelvis through the greater sciatic notch immediately caudal to the piriformis muscle. In addition to the components of the sciatic nerve, the sacral plexus also gives rise to the pudendal nerve. The pelvic splanchnic nerves (S2-4), the terminal portion of the sympathetic trunk, and the inferior hypogastric plexus all lie in close proximity to the elements of the sacral plexus.

**Approach and Technique:** The posterior superior iliac spine is identified and a line is drawn between that point and the ischial tuberosity. At a point approximately three fingerbreadths (6 cm) from the posterior superior iliac spine, an 18-gauge, 150-mm insulated Tuohy needle (Contiplex Insulated Tuohy Needle Set, B. Braun/McGaw, Medical, Inc., Bethlehem, PA) is inserted and advanced in a sagittal plane **(Fig. 1)**. The needle is walked off the contour of the greater sciatic notch into the pelvis. A brisk motor response at the ankle is sought with the aid of a peripheral nerve stimulator **(Fig. 2)**. Once a motor response is elicited at 0.2 mA (Digistim II, Neurotechnology, Houston, TX), 30 ml of local anesthetic is injected. Then, a 20-gauge epidural catheter is threaded into a fascial plane for continuous infusion of local anesthetic at a rate of 8 ml/hr.

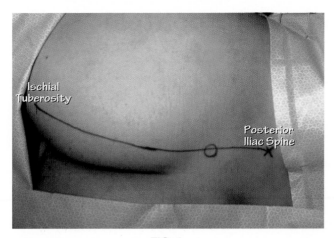

FIG. 1.

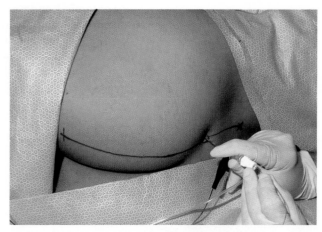

FIG. 2.

## TIP

Continuous parasacral infusion can provide excellent analgesia in the sciatic, obturator, and pudendal territories, allowing early postoperative ambulation yet avoiding problems such as urinary retention, hypotension, and bilateral limb weakness.

## SUGGESTED READINGS

Morris GF, Lang SA, Dust WN, Van der Wal M. The parasacral sciatic nerve block. *Reg Anesth* 1997;22:223–228.

Morris GF, Lang SA. Continuous parasacral sciatic nerve block: two case reports. *Reg Anesth* 1997;22:469–472.

# B. Posterior Popliteal Approach

## F. Kayser Enneking

**Patient Position:** Prone.

**Indications:** Lower leg, ankle, and foot surgery and postoperative analgesia.

**Needle Size:** 18-gauge, 50-mm insulated Tuohy needle and 20-gauge epidural catheter (Contiplex Insulated Tuohy Needle Set, B. Braun/McGaw Medical, Inc.).

**Volume:** 40 ml for initial block followed by an infusion of 4 to 8 ml/hr.

**Anatomic Landmarks:** Same as for the single-injection technique **(Fig. 3).**

**Approach and Technique:** The needle is introduced at a 60-degree angle to the skin to facilitate introduction of the catheter. After the appropriate movement in the foot has been elicited, usually inversion and dorsiflexion, the stylet is removed. Thirty to 40 ml of local anesthetic solution is given through the needle. The catheter is threaded at least 5 cm past the needle and then secured **(Fig. 4).**

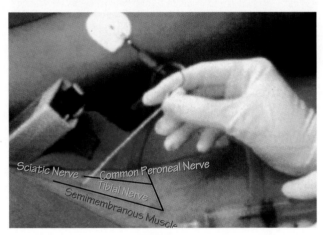

**FIG. 3.**

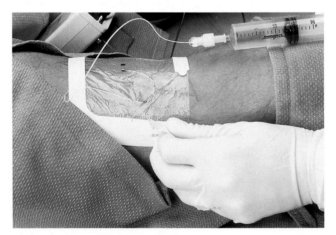

**FIG. 4.**

## TIPS

1. If the block seems slow to develop, additional local anesthetic can be given through the catheter 15 minutes after the first injection to speed onset.
2. The highest degree of success with this block occurs when inversion of the foot is noted during stimulation.
3. If the patient is going home the day of surgery, a long-lasting local anesthetic bolus can be given before removal of the catheter for prolonged analgesia. The patient must have orders for and understand the concept of nonweight bearing.

## SUGGESTED READINGS

Benzon HT, Kim C, Benzon HP, et al. Correlation between evoked motor response of the sciatic nerve and sensory blockade. *Anesthesiology* 1997;87:547–552.

Fischer HB, Peters TM, Fleming IM, Else TA. Peripheral nerve catheterization in the management of terminal cancer pain. *Reg Anesth* 1996;21:482–485.

Singelyn FJ, Aye F, Gouverneur JM. Continuous popliteal sciatic nerve block: an original technique to provide postoperative analgesia after foot surgery. *Anesth Analg* 1997;84:383–386.

# C. Lateral Popliteal Approach

## Olivier Choquet, Philippe Macaire, and Jean Louis Feugeas

**Patient Position:** Supine with the leg slightly flexed at the knee joint and placed on a pillow, and the long axis of the foot positioned at a 90-degree angle relative to the table.

**Indications:** Surgical block—this approach allows for block of the common peroneal or tibial nerve, or both, depending on the surgical requirements. Postoperative analgesia—provides prolonged analgesia of the foot and leg, at and below the knee in the territory of the sciatic nerve or the tibial and common peroneal nerves.

**Needle:** 18-gauge, 100-mm insulated Tuohy needle and 20-gauge, 100-cm epidural catheter (Contiplex Insulated Tuohy Needle Set, B. Braun/McGaw Medical, Inc.).

**Volume:** For surgical block: 10 to 15 ml of local anesthetic solution for each nerve, followed by 5 to 7 ml/hr. For postoperative analgesia: 20 ml of anesthetic solution followed by 3 to 5 ml/hr.

**Anatomic Landmarks:** The sciatic nerve runs down the posterior aspect of the thigh and divides into the tibial and common peroneal nerves in the popliteal fossa. In the popliteal fossa, the common peroneal nerve courses in a lateral direction, whereas the tibial nerve, the largest of the two, remains in the middle. In some cases, the common peroneal nerve is located several centimeters distant from the tibial nerve, and each branch is surrounded by its own fascia.

**Approach and Technique:** The groove between the biceps femoris and the vastus lateralis muscle is palpated and drawn on the skin **(Fig. 5)**. A horizontal line is drawn on the upper edge of the patella. The puncture site is the intersection of the intermuscular groove with this line. After skin preparation, the Tuohy insulated needle, connected to a nerve stimulator, is inserted 30 degrees posterior to the horizontal plane with a 45-degree cephalad direction **(Fig. 6)**. The common peroneal nerve is most often identified first **(Figs. 7, 8)**.

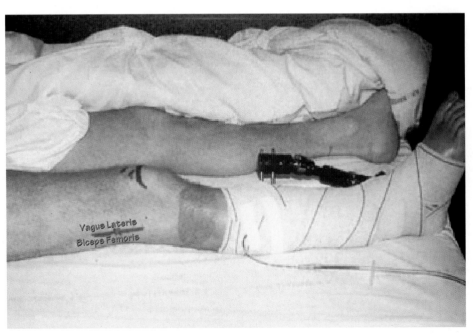

**FIG. 5.**

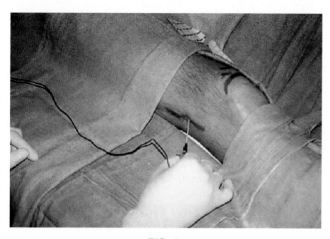

FIG. 6.

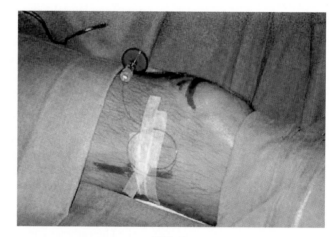

FIG. 7.

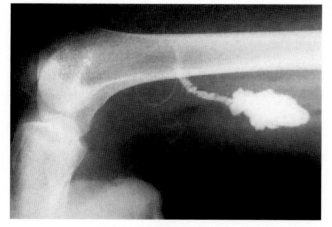

FIG. 8.

*Surgical Analgesia:* The initial current is set at between 1 and 2.5 mA (1 Hz, 100 μsec). Stimulation of the common peroneal nerve produces dorsiflexion inversion of the foot. After the nerve has been identified, the current is decreased to 0.5 mA or less to confirm the appropriate position of the needle. After negative blood aspiration, the local anesthetic solution is injected. The needle is then directed deeper (0.5 to 2 cm), following the same axis or a slightly anterior angulation to locate the tibial nerve, after increasing the current to 2.5 mA (1 Hz, 100 msec). Stimulation of the tibial nerve results in plantarflexion or inversion of the foot. The proper positioning of the needle is confirmed by maintaining the motor response with a current of less than 1 mA. When appropriate, 10 to 15 ml of local anesthetic solution is injected after negative blood aspiration. The Tuohy needle is withdrawn by 0.5 cm and 5 to 20 ml of anesthetic solution is injected before threading the catheter.

*Postoperative Analgesia:* The Tuohy needle is inserted 7 cm or more cephalad to the tip of the lateral femoral epicondyle to approach the origin of the division of the sciatic nerve. The Tuohy needle is then directed toward the nerve that predominantly innervates the surgical area. After proper identification, 20 ml of local anesthetic solution is injected and the catheter is inserted 1 to 2 cm into the nerve sheath.

## TIPS

1. Individual block of the common peroneal and tibial nerves allows faster onset.
2. If the sciatic nerve is not stimulated at the first attempt at a depth of 60 to 70 mm, the needle is withdrawn and reinserted through the same skin puncture, first 5 to 10 degrees anterior and then 5 to 10 degrees posterior relative to the initial insertion (30-degree) plane.
3. The performance of this block can be facilitated by rotating the leg slightly medially.
4. The catheter can be left in place for 3 to 4 days.
5. If the femur is contacted, the needle should be withdrawn with an additional 5 to 10 degrees of posterior angulation.
6. Local contraction of the biceps femoris muscle is observed during needle advancement. Further advancement of the needle 5 mm after cessation of local contraction of the biceps femoris muscle usually permits the operator to locate the common peroneal nerve.
7. Sensory and motor blockade is complete within 25 minutes with 1% mepivacaine; 20 ml of 0.25% to 0.375% bupivacaine with epinephrine and clonidine is sufficient for postoperative analgesia lasting 16 to 20 hours. Infusion of 0.125% to 0.25% bupivacaine or 0.2% ropivicaine through a catheter (3 to 5 ml/hr) provides excellent postoperative analgesia for 24 to 72 hours.

## SUGGESTED READINGS

Lévecque JP, Lagdanous JF, Saïssy JM. Analgésie par block continu du nerf tibial après ischémie et amputation. *Ann Fr Anesth Réanim* 1997;16:1047–1048.

Singelyn FJ, Aye F, Gouverneur JM. Continuous popliteal sciatic nerve block: an original technique to provide postoperative analgesia after foot surgery. *Anesth Analg* 1997;84:383–386.

Zetlaoui PZ, Bouaziz H. Lateral approach to the sciatic nerve in the popliteal fossa. *Anesth Analg* 1998;87:79–82.

# 25

# Continuous Femoral, Obturator, and Lateral Femoral Cutaneous Blocks

# A. Continuous Psoas Compartment (Lumbar Plexus) Block

## F. Kayser Enneking

**Patient Position:** Lateral with the operative side up.

**Indications:** When combined with a sciatic nerve block, this block provides surgical anesthesia to the lower extremity. Alone, this block provides postoperative analgesia after operations of the hip, thigh, and knee.

**Needle Size:** 18-gauge, 150-mm insulated Tuohy needle and 20-gauge epidural catheter (Contiplex Insulated Tuohy Needle Set, B. Braun/McGaw Medical, Inc., Bethlehem, PA).

**Volume:** 20 ml initially, followed by an infusion of 6 to 8 ml/hr.

**Anatomic Landmarks:** The iliac crest and the spinous process of L4. The needle entry is 5 cm lateral to the L4 spinous process and 3 mm caudal **(Fig. 1).**

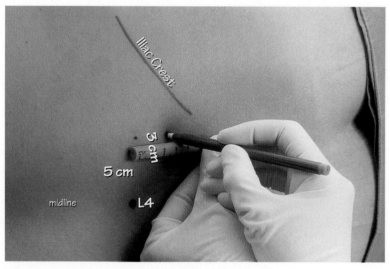

**FIG. 1.**

**Approach and Technique:** The needle is positioned perpendicular to the skin and then introduced slightly toward the midline. The transverse process of L5 is encountered. The needle is then walked cephalad off the transverse process until quadriceps motion is detected. The local anesthetic is injected and the catheter is threaded 3 to 5 ml. The catheter is aspirated and then additional local anesthetic is injected to ensure patency of the catheter **(Fig. 2).**

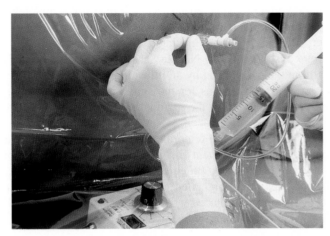

**FIG. 2.**

## TIPS

1. The operator must be aware of the possibility of epidural spread, particularly if extra local anesthetic is given. Usually this resolves uneventfully, and is not a problem with continuous low-rate infusions.
2. This block is a good alternative to central neural blockade for patients who will be anticoagulated after surgery. A retroperitoneal hematoma is not as disastrous as an epidural hematoma.
3. This block can be done as a single-injection technique, but only 20 ml should be used or epidural spread will result.
4. A stimulating needle is essential for this block. It was initially described with a loss-of-resistance technique, but was not considered a very predictable block.
5. It is important to do this block in the L4-5 interspace. Renal hematomas have been described with this block at a higher interspace.

## SUGGESTED READINGS

Aida S, Takahashi H, Shimoji K. Renal subcapsular hematoma after lumbar plexus block. *Anesthesiology* 1996;84:452–455.
Chayen D, Nathan H, Chayen M. The psoas compartment block. *Anesthesiology* 1976;45:95–99.
White IW, Chappell WA. Anaesthesia for surgical correction of fractured femoral neck: a comparison of three techniques. *Anaesthesia* 1980;35:1107–1110.

# B. Continuous Femoral Block

## F. Kayser Enneking

**Patient Position:** Supine.

**Indications:** Continuous femoral nerve block works well for postoperative analgesia in patients undergoing thigh and knee surgery. It does not completely cover an incision extending onto the tibia, but provides significant analgesia.

**Needle Size:** 18-gauge, 50-mm insulated Tuohy needle and 20-gauge epidural catheter (Contiplex Insulated Tuohy Needle Set, B. Braun/McGaw Medical, Inc.).

**Volume:** 20 ml initially, followed by an infusion of 8 to 12 ml/hr.

**Anatomic Landmarks:** Same as for the single-injection technique; however, the needle entry point is 2.5 cm below the inguinal ligament to allow a flatter needle trajectory.

**Approach and Technique:** The femoral artery is identified. The needle entry site is 2.5 cm below the inguinal ligament and 1 to 2 cm lateral to the femoral pulse. The needle is advanced cephalad at a 60-degree angle to the skin **(Fig. 3).** In almost all cases, two distinct pops are appreciated as the needle passes through thick fascial planes. The needle is correctly placed when patellar ascension is noted. The catheter is then threaded as far as it can easily be advanced **(Fig. 4).**

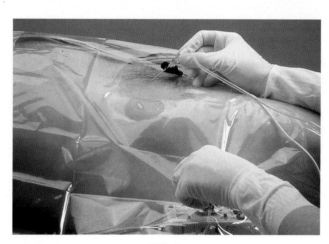

FIG. 3.

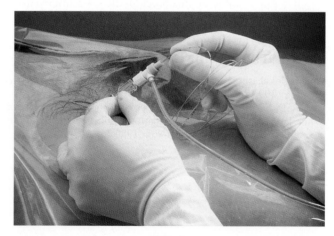

FIG. 4.

## TIPS

1. The further the catheter is threaded, the more likely the obturator and lateral femoral cutaneous nerves will be blocked as well.
2. If the medial thigh is twitching, direct the needle more laterally and at a shallower angle.
3. If the catheter does not thread easily, drop the angle of the needle so it is at a less acute angle.
4. Placing the stimulator under a clear drape allows one person to run the stimulator and drive the needle at the same time.

## SUGGESTED READINGS

Edkin BS, Spindler KP, Flanagan JF. Femoral nerve block as an alternative to parenteral narcotics for pain control after anterior cruciate ligament reconstruction. *Arthroscopy* 1995;11:404–409.

Griffith JP, Whiteley S, Gougj MJ. Prospective randomized study of a new method of providing postoperative pain relief following femoropopliteal bypass. *Br J Surg* 1996;83:1735–1738.

Mansour NY, Bennetts FE. An observational study of combined continuous lumbar plexus and single-shot sciatic nerve blocks for post-knee surgery analgesia. *Reg Anesth* 1996;21:287–291.

Schultz P, Anker-Moller E, Dahl JB, et al. Postoperative pain treatment after open knee surgery: continuous lumbar plexus block with bupivacaine versus epidural morphine. *Reg Anesth* 1991;16: 34–37.

# 26

# Continuous Nerve Sheath Blocks

F. Kayser Enneking

**Patient Position:** Varies, depending on the operation.

**Indications:** Visualization of an unblocked nerve that is likely to give rise to postoperative pain. Amputations of the extremities.

**Equipment:** Continuous epidural catheter kit opened under sterile conditions on the operative field.

**Volume:** 20 ml initially, followed by an infusion of 4 to 12 ml/hr.

**Anatomic Landmarks:** The surgeon places the catheter directly alongside the nerve under any fascial investments.

**Approach and Technique:** This block is done under direct visualization of the nerve. The surgeon makes a separate stab wound using the epidural needle to introduce the catheter into the wound. The catheter is then gently directed along the nerve under its fascial investments as far as it will easily thread, usually approximately 4 cm. The catheter is then sutured at the skin exit. After closure of the wound, the catheter is injected with 20 ml of local anesthetic and an infusion is started as soon as feasible.

## TIPS

1. Do not inject the catheter until the wound has been approximated, or the local anesthetic will be lost down the path of least resistance. Make sure any drains are crimped off during the initial injection of the local anesthetic.

2. The surgeon must be aware of the volume being placed into the wound because most of it will come out the drain. If the wound is not drained, start the infusion at the lowest rate.

3. If more than one nerve is identified, as in an upper extremity amputation, consider putting a catheter in each nerve. Pressure paresthesias can occur if a large volume of local anesthetic is administered through a single catheter.

4. For lower extremity amputations, the surgeon will see the sciatic nerve, but not the femoral nerve. The anesthesiologist should conduct a percutaneously placed continuous femoral block.

5. Give the patient access to sedatives or narcotics. The local anesthetic will take care of most of the wound pain, but the patient frequently becomes fixated on other pains and distractions. This is similar to the "hot spot" sometimes seen during a labor epidural.

6. Do not limit this technique to amputations. If the anesthesiologist could not do a percutaneous block, and the surgeon can see the nerve, the surgeon should thread a catheter.

## SUGGESTED READINGS

Enneking FK, Scarborough MT, Radson EA. Local anesthetic infusion through nerve sheath catheters for analgesia following upper extremity amputation: clinical report. *Reg Anesth* 1997; 22:351–356.

Malawer MM, Buch R, Khurana JS, Garvey T, Rice L. Postoperative infusional continuous regional analgesia: a technique for relief of postoperative pain following major extremity surgery. *Clin Orthop* 1991;266:227–237.

# SECTION IV
# Pediatric Peripheral Blocks

# 27

# Contraindications, Side Effects, and Complications of Pediatric Peripheral Blocks

Philippe Carré, Louise Gouyet, and
Claude Ecoffey

Pediatric regional anesthesia techniques have undergone great improvement in recent years. These techniques are a safe means of obtaining excellent analgesia. In addition to central blocks and, particularly, caudal anesthesia, the most frequently used regional techniques in pediatric anesthesia are peripheral blocks, which have taken on a larger role. They are usually combined with general anesthesia, but in either case, the benefit/risk ratio is always favorable because they combine efficiency, viability, and safety.

Pediatric techniques differ from those used in adults, mostly because of their pharmacologic and anatomic characteristics, but also because of the anesthesiologist–pediatric patient relationship.

The first part of this section reviews the physiologic and pharmacologic data specific to children and the safety precautions required for performing regional blocks in children. The second and third parts describe the locoregional blocks suitable for use in pediatric anesthesia. The presentation of each technique is uniform. Photographs aid in memorizing the anatomic landmarks as well as the equipment used.

## INDICATIONS

Peripheral blocks in children produce rapid and long-lasting analgesia. They facilitate examination, mobilization, and transportation (e.g., femoral nerve block for femoral fracture) or emergency treatment (surrounding wounds). Peripheral blocks are an alternative to general anesthesia when general anesthesia represents a risk (e.g., full stomach, difficult intubation, high-risk patients). They are indicated for intraoperative analgesia but also for postoperative analgesia, for which regional anesthesia is very effective and long lasting, and they constitute a viable supplementary means of handling chronic pain.

Alone or combined with sedation or general anesthesia, peripheral blocks are widely used for ambulatory surgery, such as distal surgery, removal of foreign material, superficial biopsies, fractures of the limbs, and circumcision. In these cases, they offer the advantage of good postoperative analgesia, quick recovery, and absence of residual sedation or nausea or vomiting. Their drawbacks are essentially the risk of technical failure and the persistence of a motor block.

The use of peripheral blocks leads to a reduction of the depth of anesthesia during surgery, and also necessitates morphine for postoperative analgesia and prolonged controlled ventilation in newborn or infant surgery cases.

*Systemic toxicity* of local anesthetics is the most harmful side effect and may occur after inadvertent intravascular or intraosseous injection or after overdose or prolonged infusion. Treatment and clinical symptoms of an overdose are the same as in adult patients.

In an unmedicated, conscious child, minor initial symptoms of *central nervous system toxicity* may include somnolence, headache, logorrhea, dizziness, vertigo, and perioral or lingual paresthesia. Generalized convulsions are treated with intubation and oxygenation after intravenous injection of thiopental (5 mg/kg) and 2 mg/kg succinylcholine (Burroughs Wellcome Co., Research Triangle Park, NC). If the convulsions are not stopped, an anticonvulsant (e.g., phenytoin) should be administered at the dose of 5 mg/kg over 30 minutes.

Cardiovascular toxicity can produce hypotension, cardiac arrhythmia, ventricular fibrillation, bradycardia, or even cardiac arrest. Treatment includes cardiac massage,

oxygenation, inotropic supports, and alkalinization. Tachycardia and ventricular fib-
rillations may warrant emergency electrocardioversion (3 to 6 J/kg), which can be
combined with a 5 mg/kg bretylium tosylate injection (Elkins-Sinn, Inc., Cherry
Hill, NJ).

## ADJUVANT-RELATED COMPLICATIONS

Epinephrine-related complications are local vasoconstriction and, after inadvertent
vascular injection, ventricular arrhythmia.

Epinephrine as an additive is usually recommended in pediatric anesthesia except in
cases of nerve blocks in areas where the regional blood supply is provided by terminal arteries (digital or penile block) or where there is poor blood flow (traumatic limb
ischemia) after short surgical procedures.

Less than 2 μg/kg clonidine in children does not induce any hemodynamic side
effects. However, clonidine-induced sedation can delay recovery.

Prolonged motor or sensory blockade can lead to skin necrosis. Methemoglobinemia has been described with the use of EMLA® cream (Astra Pharmaceutical Products, Inc., Westborough, MA) in infants. Allergic reactions to local anesthetics have
not been described in children. It is essential to have thorough knowledge of the indications, contraindications, advantages, and complications of regional anesthesia.

The benefit/risk ratio is excellent, especially for certain blocks: femoral, iliofascial,
axillary, and penile. The regional blocks described in the following chapters require
complete knowledge of the anatomic landmarks involved. Training in the use of these
blocks should be supervised by specialists in pediatric anesthesiology.

# 28

# General Considerations
# for Pediatric Blocks

Philippe Carré, Louise Gouyet, and
Claude Ecoffey

## ANATOMY

Myelination begins during the fetal period and continues to the age of 3 years. In infants, the fiber diameter is smaller, the myelin sheath thinner, and the internodal distance smaller, so lower concentrations of local anesthetics are required to produce block, leading to fewer toxic effects. Local distribution is excellent because of several factors, including volume, concentration, and the presence and thickness of the aponeuroses and sheaths surrounding the nerves. The block takes effect more rapidly, but its duration is shorter.

## PHARMACOLOGY

Local distribution and systemic absorption are greater in young children because their cardiac output and regional blood flow are higher. The free amount of local anesthetic is higher in the newborn because of lower levels of albumin and $\alpha_1$-acid-glycoprotein. The plasma concentration of glycoprotein increases gradually with age, reaching adult levels at 9 months of age. The free amount of local anesthetic is inversely related to the concentrations of plasma protein. Before 3 months of age, lidocaine, because of its weaker protein binding, the lesser influence of age on its free plasma fraction, and its lower systemic toxicity, is sometimes preferred to bupivacaine.

## PSYCHOLOGY

It is unacceptable for a child to suffer needlessly or to impose on a child a physically and psychologically unpleasant technique when safer and less unpleasant alternatives are available. The anesthesiologist should explain to the child and his or her parents the advantages of performing regional anesthesia, as well as the procedure and side effects, such as the possible persistence of a motor block. Anesthesiologists should also warn of the possibility of technical failure and outline alternative procedures (e.g., general anesthesia, complementary block, sedation).

The child should be premedicated before being taken to the operating room and be allowed to bring a familiar toy. In the operating room, the atmosphere should be friendly, calm, and warm. EMLA® cream (Astra Pharmaceutical Products, Inc., Westborough, MA) should be applied in the preoperative period to the possible point of puncture (intravenous access and block). It is important the child does not see the procedure. After surgery, the child should be admitted to a recovery room until sensory and motor blocks are resolved.

Regional anesthesia provides excellent postoperative analgesia that allows rapid discontinuation of the intravenous line and prompt initiation of oral fluids to be started quickly.

# 29

# Technical Considerations for Pediatric Blocks

Philippe Carré, Louise Gouyet, and
Claude Ecoffey

## EQUIPMENT

For most regional techniques, 21- to 23-gauge needles are used. The type of bevel is an important factor in the selection of a needle because trauma to the structure traversed depends on the bevel. A short bevel with a 30-degree angle is preferred for most blocks. The needle length depends on the type of block and the age and weight of the patient.

Eliciting paresthesia by means of an electrical nerve stimulator is necessary for localizing nerve trunks. It is difficult to explain the concept of paresthesia to a child younger than 8 to 9 years of age; good cooperation is difficult to achieve. The nerve stimulator should deliver electric current in 50- to 100-msec pulses, with a constant intensity adjusted between 0.2 and 5 mA, and a frequency of 1 to 5 Hz. The needle is connected to the negative pole of the generator, whereas the skin electrode is connected to the anode.

## LOCAL ANESTHETICS SOLUTIONS

The principal solutions used for pediatric regional anesthesia are bupivacaine, lidocaine, and mepivacaine. Recommended doses are shown in **Table 1**. Ropivacaine has not yet been used in pediatric regional blocks. Bupivacaine should not be used in newborns or in infants younger than 3 months of age. In general, the concentrations of local anesthetics are more diluted in children than in adults. The precise dose and concentration are based on the age and weight of the patient and nature of the block. Calculate individually for each child the maximum permissible dosage in milligrams per kilogram and the volume corresponding to the concentration of the selected local anesthetic that has to be adapted if several blocks are combined (e.g., sciatic and femoral blocks). In children up to 3 months of age, the maximum dose of lidocaine is 10 mg/kg. The dose for 0.25% bupivacaine with epinephrine is 2.5 mg/kg (1 ml/kg), and can be used in children over 3 months of age who need surgery of long duration or analgesia lasting longer than 3 hours. Mepivacaine can be used for a 6-month-old infant if a motor block and long-lasting analgesia with less toxicity than bupivacaine are needed. For a child weighing more than 40 kg, the dosage would be the same as for an adult (i.e., a maximum of 600 mg lidocaine, 600 mg mepivacaine, and 150 mg bupivacaine).

To achieve optimal anesthetic effects with pediatric blocks, local anesthetics are usually combined. In combination, the toxicity of local anesthetics is additive.

**Table 1.** *Principal local anesthetics used for pediatric peripheral blocks*

| Agent | Concentration (%) | Dose (mg/kg) | Maximum recommended doses without epinephrine (mg/kg) | Maximum recommended doses with epinephrine[a] (mg/kg) | Latency (min) | Duration (hr) |
|---|---|---|---|---|---|---|
| Lidocaine | 0.5–2 | 5 | 7.5 | 10 | 10–15 | 1–2 |
| Bupivacaine | 0.25–0.5 | 2 | 2.5 | 3 | 20–30 | 2–6 |
| Mepivacaine | 1 | 8 | 8 | — | 10–15 | 2–3 |

[a]Epinephrine is given at a concentration of 1/400,000 before 3 months of age, and 1/200,000 after 3 months age. Mepivacaine solution does not exist with epinephrine.

Vasoconstrictors, such as epinephrine, reduce systemic absorption of the local anesthetic, prolong analgesia effects, and can be useful in detecting an inadvertent intravascular injection. Epinephrine as an additive is usually recommended in pediatric anesthesia, except in cases of a nerve block in an area where regional blood supply is provided by terminal arteries (e.g., penile block). In general, the concentration recommended is 1/200,000 in children and 1/400,000 in the infant and the newborn.

$\alpha$–Adrenergic agonists such as clonidine have been used to prolong the analgesic effects of local anesthetics without any hemodynamic effects. They offer sedation in short procedures and cumulative effects if combined with epinephrine.

## RECOMMENDATIONS

*After placing an IV line*, all regional anesthesia should be performed in an area with a resuscitation cart, an electrocardiograph (ECG), and a respiratory monitor nearby.

All equipment for regional anesthesia should be stocked in a cart designed specifically for that purpose. All regional blocks are performed under aseptic conditions.

After defining anatomic landmarks, the anesthesiologist, wearing gloves, prepares the material in an aseptic manner. The puncture site is cleaned thoroughly with an antiseptic solution. Before injection, muscular contractions should be obtained for minimal intensity (<1 mA). An aspiration test should be performed before each injection. The test dose (1 ml) stops muscular contraction, and no changes should be seen on the ECG monitor for 30 to 40 seconds after the test dose.

Local anesthetic solution should be administered slowly over a period of at least 60 to 120 seconds, regardless of the type of block, with repeated aspirations for every 5 ml of injected solution.

If doubt arises over any part of the procedure, the injection should be stopped immediately (e.g., abnormal resistance, pain if the child is awake, ECG or neurologic abnormalities). After evaluation of the distribution, extension, and quality of the block by the puncture technique, surgery can begin.

Because younger children are often frightened by the operating room and cannot cooperate with the anesthesiologist, all children younger than 5 years of age receive general anesthesia combined with regional anesthesia. After 5 years of age, the child's anxiety can be reduced if the anesthesiologist has won his or her confidence by explaining the procedures. If the child prefers, general anesthesia can be used if there is no contraindication (e.g., full stomach). After induction, the regional block is performed with a higher nerve stimulator intensity (1 to 2 mA). If the child is cooperative, but slightly anxious, intravenous sedation with a benzodiazepine can be given (midazolam 0.1 mg/kg), or a 50%/50% $O_2$/$N_2O$ mixture can be administered by mask.

A detailed anesthetic record is maintained of anesthetic agents used, type of regional block performed (length of needle, dose and volume of local anesthetic solution), anesthetic drugs administrated (intravenous or local), and evaluation of the block and possible complications. The child remains in the recovery room until motor function returns, or until the Aldrete's score is over 10 in cases in which peripheral block was combined with sedation or general anesthesia.

# 30

# Parascalene Block

Philippe Carré, Louise Gouyet, and
Claude Ecoffey

**Patient Position:** Supine with the head turned away from the side to be blocked and with the arms extended along the sides of the body, and shoulders raised with a rolled sheet.

**Indications:** Recommended for elective or emergency surgery of the upper limb when lesions are located above the elbow or when the limb cannot be moved, either because of severe pain or because of the nature of the lesion. This block provides excellent intraoperative and postoperative analgesia. The lower branches of the cervical plexus are blocked in more than 50% of reported block procedures.

**Specific Contraindications:** Acute or chronic respiratory insufficiency (cystic fibrosis) or whenever the surgery mandates bilateral supraclavicular block (possibility of phrenic block).

**Side Effects:** A stellate ganglion block may occur with Horner's syndrome (ptosis of the eye, myosis, anophthalmos, hyperhemia of the conjunctivae, hyperthermia and anhidrosis of the face).

This insertion avoids the risk of damage to the vertebral artery or the large blood vessels of the neck, of a pneumothorax, or of an epidural or intrathecal injection.

**Needle Size:** 24-gauge, 25-mm b-beveled Stimuplex insulated needle (B. Braun/McGaw Medical, Inc., Bethlehem, PA).

**Volume:** 0.5 ml/kg.

**Anatomic Landmarks:** The midpoint of the clavicle and Chassaignac's tubercle (anterior tubercle of the transverse process of the sixth cervical vertebra), which is projected on the skin at the intersection of the sternocleidomastoid, with the transverse plain passing through the cricoid cartilage **(Fig. 1)**.

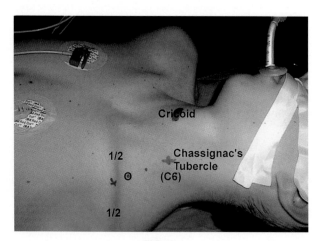

**FIG. 1.**

**Approach and Technique:** The point of puncture is situated at the junction of the upper two-thirds and lower one-third of the line joining the midpoint of the clavicle and Chassaignac's tubercle. The needle is inserted perpendicular to the skin in an anteroposterior plane, until muscle twitches are elicited **(Fig. 2).** If the needle is too lateral, muscle contractions of the shoulder are seen when the supraclavicular nerve, which lies outside the plexus, is stimulated. If the needle is too medial or too deep, the phrenic nerve may be stimulated, leading to contractions of the diaphragm. In either case, the needle should be withdrawn up to the subcutaneous tissue and redirected correctly.

**Pediatric Particularities:** The brachial plexus is located at a depth of 7 to 30 mm from the skin, depending on age. This technique gives excellent analgesia of the upper extremities and is safer and has a lower incidence of complications than other supraclavicular blocks (i.e., interscalene and perisubclavian blocks). The distal nerve block requires the cooperation of the patient, which is difficult to expect in awake children.

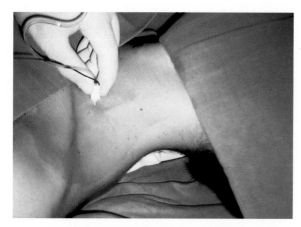

**FIG. 2.**

## SUGGESTED READINGS

Dalens B, Vanneuville G, Tanguy A. A new parascalene approach to the brachial plexus in children: comparison with the supraclavicular approach. *Anesth Analg* 1987;66:1264–1271.

Vongvises P, Panijayanond T. A parascalene technique of brachial plexus anesthesia. *Anesth Analg* 1979;58:267–273.

# 31

# Axillary Block

Philippe Carré, Louise Gouyet, and
Claude Ecoffey

**Patient Position:** Supine with the arm adducted 90 degrees to the body and forearm flexed at a right angle to the arm and supinated.

**Indications:** Elective or emergency surgery of the forearm and the hand, as well as for intraoperative or postoperative analgesia.

**Specific Contraindications:** Axillary lymphadenopathy or when the situation requires the limb to be immobilized, as with intense pain or an unstable fracture.

**Needle Size:** For patients under 30 kg, 24-gauge, 25-mm b-beveled Stimuplex insulated needle (B. Braun/McGaw Medical, Inc., Bethlehem, PA); for patients over 30 kg, 24-gauge, 50-mm b-beveled Stimuplex insulated needle (B. Braun/McGaw Medical, Inc.).

**Volume:** 0.5 mg/kg.

**Anatomic Landmarks:** Axillary artery, major pectoral muscle, coracobrachialis muscle. The point of puncture is situated at the intersection where the pectoralis major muscle crosses the coracobrachialis muscle, at the upper border of the axillary artery. A characteristic cutaneous dimple often marks this point.

**Approach and Technique:** The needle is introduced at an angle of 45 degrees at the upper margin of the axillary artery with the needle pointing toward the midpoint of the clavicle. A characteristic pop is felt as the needle enters the periplexus sheath. Axillary artery pulsations are transmitted to the needle. If a nerve stimulator is used, muscle twitches are seen in the forearm and the hand. Once the correct position of the needle is confirmed, the injection can begin **(Fig. 1)**. Several variations have been described, one of which is the Dalens' technique. The needle is introduced perpendicular to the skin surface, the arm in the direction of the upper border of the axillary artery and the humerus until the periplexus sheath is penetrated. If a tourniquet is necessary for the surgical procedure, a subcutaneous infiltration of local anesthetic solution at the puncture point may be needed to block the cutaneous medial nerve.

**Pediatric Particularities:** Near 100% success rate, high benefit/risk ratio.

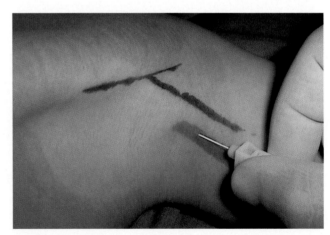

**FIG. 1.**

### SUGGESTED READING

Winnie AP, Collins VH. The subclavian perivascular technique of brachial plexus anesthesia. *Anesthesiology* 1964;25:353.

# 32

# Sciatic Nerve Blocks

Philippe Carré, Louise Gouyet, and
Claude Ecoffey

# A. Posterior Approach

**Patient Position:** The child is placed in the decubitus lateral position with the side to be blocked lying uppermost. The thighs are flexed at 120 degrees with the knees folded at 90 degrees.

**Indications:** Analgesia for trauma of the leg and foot. In elective surgery, a sciatic nerve block can be performed for surgery on the foot and combined with a femoral nerve block. All operations on the lower limb can be performed.

**Needle Size:** The following needle sizes are recommended:

- Under 10 kg, 24-gauge, 25-mm b-beveled Stimuplex insulated needle (B. Braun/McGaw Medical, Inc., Bethlehem, PA).
- Up to 25 kg, 22-gauge, 50-mm b-beveled Stimuplex insulated needle (B. Braun/McGaw Medical, Inc.).
- Over 25 kg, 21-gauge, 100-mm b-beveled Stimuplex insulated needle (B. Braun/McGaw Medical, Inc.).

**Volume:** 0.5 ml/kg. Do not use over 35 ml. When a femoral nerve block is combined with a sciatic nerve block, the total dose is reduced by one-third for each block.

**Anatomic Landmarks:** The posterosuperior iliac spine, the tip of the coccyx, the ischial tuberosity, and the greater trochanter of the femur. The point of puncture is the midpoint of the line joining the greater trochanter and the tip of the coccyx.

**Approach and Technique:** The needle is introduced slowly perpendicular to the skin, directed toward the lateral border of the ischial tuberosity, medially and upward until muscle twitches are elicited in the foot **(Fig. 1)**. Dorsiflexion of the foot and eversion (tibial nerve) or plantarflexion of the foot and an inversion (common peroneal nerve) are seen.

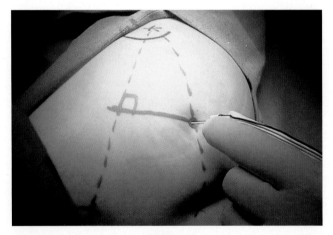

**FIG. 1.**

## PEDIATRIC PARTICULARITIES

1. The depth at which twitches are seen (between 16 and 60 mm) depends on the patient's age. Because there is a risk of injury to the sciatic nerve with this block, it should be performed by senior physicians.
2. The sciatic nerve has two characteristics:
   a. The onset of analgesia is slow (perhaps more than 30 minutes).
   b. The duration of analgesia is markedly prolonged, frequently exceeding 10 hours.

## SUGGESTED READINGS

Dalens B, Tanguy A, Vanneuville G. Sciatic nerve block in children: comparison of the posterior, anterior and lateral approaches in 180 pediatric patients. *Anesth Analg* 1990;70:131–137.
Guardini R, Waldron BA, Wallace WA. Sciatic nerve block: a new lateral approach. *Acta Anaesthesiol Scand* 1985;29:515–519.

# B. Lateral Approach

**Patient Position:** Supine with the leg slightly rotated externally, if possible.

**Indications:** Analgesia for trauma of the foot or leg. In many cases, combined with a femoral nerve block. Foot surgery (e.g., clubfoot surgery).

**Needle Size:** The following needle sizes are recommended:

- Under 10 kg, 24-gauge, 25-mm b-beveled Stimuplex insulated needle (B. Braun/McGaw Medical, Inc.).
- Up to 25 kg, 22-gauge, 50-mm b-beveled Stimuplex insulated needle (B. Braun/McGaw Medical, Inc.).
- Over 25 kg, 21-gauge, 100-mm b-beveled Stimuplex insulated needle (B. Braun/McGaw Medical, Inc.).

**Volume:** 0.5 ml/kg. Do not use over 35 ml.

**Anatomic Landmarks:** Greater trochanter.

**Approach and Technique:** The point of puncture is located on the lateral aspect of the thigh (1 to 2 cm, depending on age) below the greater trochanter. The needle is inserted perpendicular to the long axis of the limb in the horizontal plane, directed toward the position bordering the femur and the ischial tuberosity **(Fig. 2).** If the needle touches bone, it is withdrawn and reinserted more dorsally, under the femur.

**Pediatric Particularities:** The depth at which the sciatic nerve is found depends on age. Lateral sciatic nerve blocks are effective, safe, and simple. There is no need to mobilize the child.

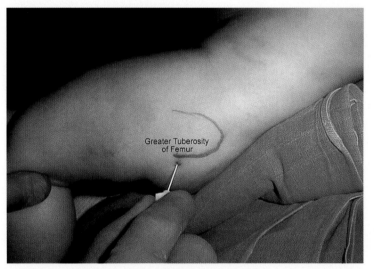

**FIG. 2.**

# C. Popliteal Approach

**Patient Position:** Prone position where the legs are flexed at approximately 30 degrees with a rolled towel beneath the ankles.

**Indications:** Foot surgery, with the exception of the medial aspect of the thigh, which is blocked with a saphenous nerve block.

**Needle Size:** 22-gauge, 50-mm b-beveled Stimuplex insulated needle (B. Braun/McGaw Medical, Inc.).

**Volume:** 0.5 ml/kg. The volume injected should be less than 35 ml. Reduce by one-third if combined with a femoral block.

**Anatomic Landmarks:** Between the tendons of the biceps femoris and the semi-tendinous, the intercondylar line, and the bisector of the angle created by the summit of the popliteal fossa.

**Approach and Technique:** The point of puncture is located 1 cm lateral to the bisector, at the junction of the upper one-third and the lower two-thirds of the segment extending from the summit of the popliteal fossa and the intercondylar line. The needle is inserted at a right angle to the posterior aspect of the popliteal fossa until muscle twitches are elicited in the flexor muscles of the foot **(Fig. 3)**.

**Pediatric Particularities:** This block should not be performed by beginners.

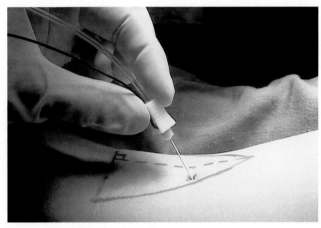

**FIG. 3.**

## SUGGESTED READING

Rorie DK, Byer DE, Nelson DO, Sittipong R, Johnson KAK. Assessment of block of the sciatic nerve in the popliteal fossa. *Anesth Analg* 1980;59:371.

# 33

# Femoral Nerve Blocks

Philippe Carré, Louise Gouyet, and
Claude Ecoffey

# A. Fascia Iliaca Compartment Block

**Patient Position:** Supine with a slight adduction of the thigh.

**Indications:** The fascia iliaca compartment block blocks the femoral nerve in all cases, and the lateral cutaneous nerve of the thigh and the obturator nerve in 75% of cases.

**Needle Size:** For patients under 25 kg, 24-gauge, 25-mm b-beveled Stimuplex insulated needle (B. Braun/McGaw Medical, Inc., Bethlehem, PA); for patients over 25 kg, 22-gauge, 50-mm b-beveled Stimuplex insulated needle (B. Braun/McGaw Medical, Inc.)

**Volume:** 0.5 ml/kg. Do not use over 30 ml.

**Anatomic Landmarks:** The ligament inguinal, which extends from the anterosuperior iliac spine to the pubic tubercle and the femoral artery.

**Approach and Technique:** The site of puncture is 0.5 to 1.0 cm below the junction of the lateral one-third and medial two-thirds of the inguinal ligament, lateral to the femoral artery. The needle is introduced at a right angle to the skin. A first loss of resistance is felt when the needle pierces the fascia lata. The second is felt as it penetrates the fascia iliaca **(Fig. 1)**.

**Pediatric Particularities:** Excellent benefit/risk ratio at any age; can be performed by beginners, but sometimes the sensation of passing the double fascia can be difficult to appreciate in small children. This block is better for postoperative analgesia than for femoral block.

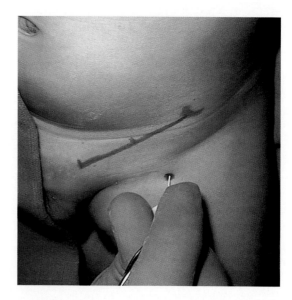

FIG. 1.

## SUGGESTED READING

Dalens B, Vanneuville G, Tanguy A. Comparison of the fascia iliaca compartment block with the 3-in-1 block in children. *Anesth Analg* 1989;69:705–713.

# B. Femoral Block

**Patient Position:** Supine with the lower limb adducted, the knees slightly flexed, and the lateral border of the feet in contact with the bed.

**Indications:** The anesthetized area will be the quadriceps group of muscles, the periosteum of the shaft of the femur, skin of the anterior aspect of the thigh, the medial part of the leg, and a small portion of the foot. Analgesia is used in cases of fracture of the femur, surgery of the thigh, and knee and leg surgery combined with a sciatic block.

**Needle Size:** For patients under 25 kg, 24-gauge, 25-mm b-beveled Stimuplex insulated needle (B. Braun/McGaw Medical, Inc.). For patients over 25 kg, 22-gauge, 50-mm b-beveled Stimuplex insulated needle (B. Braun/McGaw Medical, Inc.).

**Volume:** 0.5 ml/kg. Do not use over 35 ml.

**Anatomic Landmarks:** Inguinal ligament, which extends from the anterosuperior iliac spine to the pubic tubercle, and the femoral artery, which can be palpated just below the inguinal ligament **(Fig. 2).**

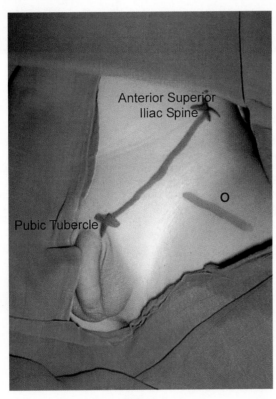

**FIG. 2.**

**Approach and Technique:** The site of puncture is 0.5 to 1.0 cm below the inguinal ligament and lateral to the femoral artery. The needle is inserted perpendicularly into the skin surface or with a slight upward tilt until muscle twitches of the rectus femoris are seen **(Fig. 3).**

**Pediatric Particularities:** Success rate is near 100%; has a very good benefit/risk ratio; can be performed by beginners; should be proposed for any fracture of the femur and for any age.

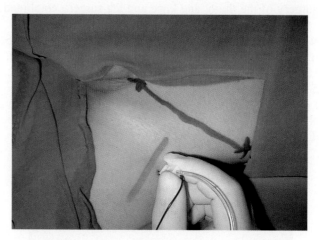

**FIG. 3.**

## SUGGESTED READINGS

Khoo ST, Brown TCK. Femoral nerve block: the anatomical basis for a single injection technique. *Anaesth Intensive Care* 1983;11:40.

McNicol LR. Lower limb blocks for children. Lateral cutaneous and femoral nerve blocks for postoperative pain relief in paediatric practice. *Anaesthesia* 1986;41:27–31.

Ronchi L, Rosenbaum D, Athouel A, et al. Femoral nerve blockade in children using bupivacaine. *Anesthesiology* 1989;70:622–624.

# 34

# Ankle Block

Philippe Carré, Louise Gouyet, and
Claude Ecoffey

**Patient Position:** Dorsal decubitus with the leg flexed at 45 degrees with slight external rotation for the tibial nerve and with the foot resting on its lateral border for the saphenous nerve.

**Indications:** Surgery of the leg and foot because the saphenous nerve, which is a terminal branch of the femoral nerve, provides sensory innervation to the distal part of the lower limb.

**Needle Size:** 22-gauge, 50-mm b-beveled Stimuplex insulated needle (B. Braun/McGaw Medical, Inc., Bethlehem, PA).

**Volume:** 2 to 4 ml for common peroneal nerve block; 6 to 8 ml for the tibial nerve block.

**Anatomic Landmarks:** The foot can be blocked with four punctures; the dorsum of the foot is innervated by the saphenous nerve for the inside and both the superficial and deep peroneal nerves for the outside, whereas the sole is essentially supplied by the terminal branches of the tibial nerve. The lateral aspect of the foot is supplied by the sural nerve. Anatomic landmarks are the lateral and medial malleolus, the Achilles tendon, and the neck of the fibula. The ankle block is obtained after blocking the tibial nerve, the common peroneal nerve, the saphenous nerve, and the sural nerve.

**Approach and Technique:** The first nerve to be blocked is the tibial nerve. The point of puncture is located above the medial malleolus, just lateral to the Achilles tendon. The needle is introduced at right angles to the skin up to a point where twitches are noted in the foot (plantarflexion of the toes; **Fig. 1**).

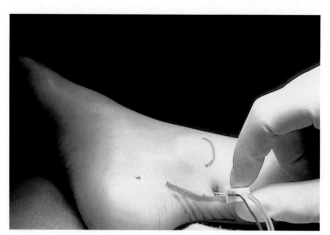

**FIG.1.**

The point of puncture for the common peroneal nerve block is the neck of the fibula. The needle is inserted perpendicularly and horizontally until dorsal flexion of the toes and eversion are noted.

The saphenous nerve is blocked by a subcutaneous injection administered along a circular line drawn around the ankle at approximately 2 cm above the medial malleolus.

The sural nerve is blocked in the same manner as the saphenous nerve, but on the lateral malleolus.

**Pediatric Particularities:** A nerve stimulator should be used for the common peroneal nerve block and should be avoided in small children (weight <20 kg), especially if general anesthesia is combined. No complications have been ascribed to this technique, but the nerve is vulnerable at the fibular neck (superficially attached to the bone) and inadequate positioning can occur, causing damage to the nerve by compression.

## SUGGESTED READING

Schurman DJ. Ankle-block anesthesia for foot surgery. *Anesthesiology* 1976;44:348–352.

# 35

# Penile Block

Philippe Carré, Louise Gouyet, and
Claude Ecoffey

**Patient Position:** Supine position.

**Indications:** Surgery of the foreskin (phimosis, paraphimosis, circumcision), postoperative analgesia after repair of hypospadias.

**Needle Size:** 22-gauge, 30-mm spinal needle.

**Volume:** 0.1 ml/kg for each side with 0.5% bupivacaine without epinephrine. Epinephrine is absolutely contraindicated because it can lead to a spasm of the dorsal arteries of the penis with subsequent ischemia and necrosis of the gland.

**Anatomic Landmarks:** Pubic symphysis.

**Approach and Technique:** After pulling the penis gently downward and identifying the pubic symphysis, the two points are marked just below each pubic rami approximately 0.5 to 1.0 cm on either side of the pubic symphysis. The needle is introduced at the puncture site, perpendicular to the skin. Penetration is stopped in the subpubic space after a distinct elastic recoil is felt, corresponding to the crossing of the deep membranous layer of the superficial fascia **(Fig. 1).** The same procedure is repeated on the opposite side.

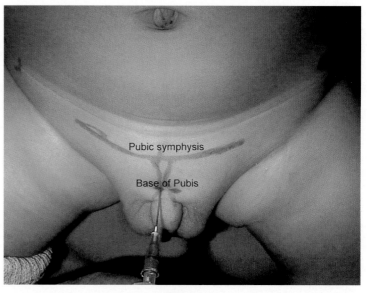

**FIG. 1.**

**Pediatric Particularities:** The depth of insertion correlates with age (8 mm for a newborn, 30 mm for a young adult). The old technique of midline puncture can injure the dorsal artery of the penis, leading to a compressive hematoma, possibly resulting in glans necrosis. The penile block is an effective, safe technique and easy to perform, even for beginners. Analgesia obtained by this block lasts for at least 24 hours.

For any operation on the foreskin, a penile block is the procedure of choice, preferable to a caudal epidural (less morbidity), the performance of a ring block at the base of the penis (20% inconsistent results), or a local application of lidocaine gel or EMLA® cream, which produce less postoperative analgesia.

## SUGGESTED READING

Dalens B, Vanneuville G, Dechelott P. Penile block via the subpubic space in 100 children. *Anesth Analg* 1989;69:41–45.

# 36

# Ilioinguinal Block

Philippe Carré, Louise Gouyet, and
Claude Ecoffey

**Patient Position:** Supine position.
**Indications:** Hernia repair.
**Needle:** 22-gauge, 30-mm spinal needle.
**Volume:** 0.4 ml/kg with 0.5 % bupivacaine without epinephrine.
**Anatomic Landmarks:** Anterior superior iliac spine **(Fig. 1).**

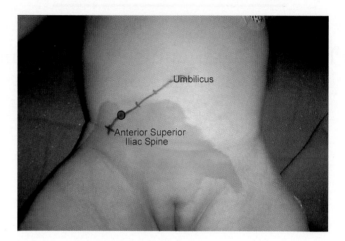

FIG. 1.

**Approach and Technique:** A short-bevel needle is inserted just below and medial to the anterosuperior iliac spine. Depending on the size of the patient, the distance is 0.5 cm in the infant and 2 cm in the adolescent. The needle is slowly advanced until there is a loss of resistance, which occurs as the aponeurosis of the external oblique muscle is pierced. The needle is then orientated in the direction of the middle of the inguinal ligament, and then the injection can begin **(Fig. 2).**

**Pediatric Particularities:** This block represents an alternative with less morbidity than the caudal block for hernia repair.

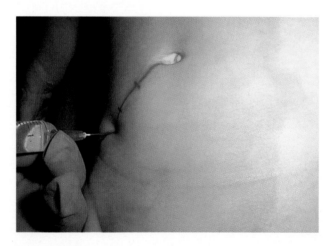

FIG. 2.

## SUGGESTED READING

Hinkle AJ. Percutaneous inguinal block for the outpatient management of post-herniorrhaphy pain in pediatric ambulatory surgery. *Anesthesiology* 1987;67:411–413.

# Subject Index

**B**

B-beveled insulated needles, 9, 9f
  in axillary blocks, 22, 22f, 41, 41f
  in femoral blocks, 97, 97f
  in lower extremity blocks, 64
  peripheral, 8, 8f
    in sciatic nerve blocks, 72
  in posterior lumbar plexus (psoas)
      blocks, 90–91
  in sciatic nerve blocks, 76, 76f, 82, 87
  in supraclavicular blocks, 37
  in truncular blocks, 47–48
  in ulnar blocks, 51–52, 51f 52f
  in wrist blocks, 56, 56f
Beck's anterior approach
  of sciatic nerve, 65, 81, 82f
Benzodiazepines
  in cervical blocks, 110
  in pediatric peripheral blocks, 187
Bier blocks, 122–123
  anatomic landmarks, 122
  approach and technique, 122, 122f
  indications for, 122
  patient position, 122
  toxicity of, 123
Blood aspiration
  in superior laryngeal nerve block, 130
Brachial plexus
  in axillary blocks, 22, 22f
  in continuous interscalene block, 145
  in infraclavicular block, 21, 21f
  innervation of, 19f
  in interscalene block, 20, 20f
  nerves of
    anastomosis between, 18, 18t
  in parascalene block, 191
  in subclavicular block, 21, 21f
  tangential access to
    in supraclavicular block, 21, 21f
Brachial plexus blocks
  anatomic considerations for, 18–19
  extension of, 19–24
  median nerve in, 19f, 21
  musculocutaneous nerve in, 19f
  radial nerve in, 19f
  surgical indications for, 25–27
  ulnar nerve in, 19f, 21
Bronchoscopy
  superior laryngeal nerve block for,
      130
Bunionectomy, 66t
Bupivacaine, 26–27
  in cervical blocks, 109
  in continuous peripheral blocks, 140,
      141
  in humeral blocks, 26–27
  in ilioinguinal blocks, 214
  in intercostal blocks, 118
  in pediatric peripheral blocks, 186
  in penile blocks, 211
  in peribulbar blocks, 112

  in sciatic nerve blocks, 82, 88
  in thoracic paravertebral blocks, 135
  toxicity of, 12

**C**

Calcaneal nerve, 64f
  in foot, 103f
Calf
  lateral cutaneous nerve in, 103f
Cardiovascular system
  toxic effects on
    of local anesthesia, 12
    of pediatric peripheral blocks,
        180–181
Carotid endarterectomy
  cervical block for, 108
Carpal tunnel syndrome
  musculocutaneous nerve blocks for, 26t
Cataracts
  surgery of
    peribulbar blocks for, 112
Catheters
  in continuous wrist block, 156, 160–161
  dislodgment of
    in continuous interscalene block, 145
  in fascia iliacus block, 94
  for nerve stimulation, 9–10, 9f
  in subclavicular blocks, 25
  threading of
    in continuous axillary block, 153
    in continuous femoral block, 173
    in continuous infraclavicular block,
        150
Central nervous system
  toxic effects on
    of cervical blocks, 110
    of interscalene blocks, 32
    of local anesthesia, 12
    of pediatric peripheral blocks, 180
    of peribulbar blocks, 114
Central neural blockade
  alternative to
    in postoperative anticoagulation,
        171
Cerebral ischemia
  in cervical block, 110
Cervical block, 108–110
  anatomic landmarks, 108, 108f
  approach and technique, 109–110
    deep, 109, 109f
    superficial, 110
  indications for, 108
  needles, 108
  patient position, 108
  sedation for, 110
  side effects of, 110
  volume, 108
Chassaignac's tubercle
  and parascalene block, 190, 191
Chelly's anterior approach
  of sciatic nerve, 65, 79f, 82, 82f

Chloroprocaine
  in lower extremity blocks, 69
Cholecystectomy
  pain from
    thoracic paravertebral block for, 134
Circumcision
  penile block for, 211
Clonidine, 13
  in cervical blocks, 110
  in continuous peripheral blocks, 141
  in continuous wrist blocks, 156
  in pediatric peripheral blocks, 181, 187
  in peribulbar blocks, 115
  side effects of, 13, 181
Coagulopathy, 4
Cocaine
  in airway blocks, 126
Colles fracture
  axillary blocks for, 26t
Common peroneal nerve, 64f, 65
  in ankle blocks, 207
  in continuous sciatic blocks
    lateral popliteal approach, 166, 167f
  in sciatic nerve blocks, 72, 73f
Compression syndrome
  after total knee replacement, 68
Conjunctiva
  surgery of
    peribulbar blocks for, 112
Continuous axillary blocks, 152, 152f
Continuous brachial plexus set, 9, 9f
Continuous cutaneous blocks, 170–173
  femoral, 172–173
  psoas compartment (lumbar plexus),
      170–171
Continuous femoral blocks, 172–173, 172f
Continuous infraclavicular blocks,
      148–150
  anatomic landmarks, 148, 148f
  approach and technique, 149, 149f
  indications for, 148
Continuous interscalene block, 144–145
  anatomic landmarks, 144
  approach and technique, 144, 144f
  indications for, 144
  patient position, 144
  side effects of, 145
Continuous lumbar plexus block
  for total knee replacement, 66t
Continuous nerve sheath blocks, 176
Continuous peripheral blocks, 140–176
  axillary, 152–153
  catheter placement
    guidelines, 140
  femoral cutaneous, 170–173
  infraclavicular, 148–150
  interscalene, 144–145
  local anesthesia for, 141
    toxicity of, 141
  nerve sheath, 176
  sciatic, 156–168

wrist, 156–160
Continuous psoas compartment (lumbar
        plexus) block, 170–171
    anatomic landmarks, 170, 170f
    approach and technique, 171, 171f
    indications for, 170
    patient position, 170
Continuous regional anesthesia. See
        Continuous peripheral blocks
Continuous sciatic blocks
    anatomic landmarks, 162, 164, 164f,
        166
    approach and technique, 162–164, 166,
        166f–167f
    indications for, 162, 164, 166
    lateral popliteal approach, 162, 164,
        166–168
    motor response
        of ankle, 162
    needles, 162, 164, 166
    parasacral approach, 162–163
    patient position, 162, 164, 166
    posterior popliteal approach, 164–165
    postoperative analgesia, 168
    surgical analgesia, 168
    volume
        lateral popliteal approach, 162, 164,
            166
        posterior popliteal approach, 164
Continuous wrist blocks, 156–160
    anatomic landmarks, 156
    approach and technique, 156–160,
        157f–159f
    indications for, 156
    patient position, 156
Convulsions
    in pediatric peripheral blocks, 180
Cricothyroid membrane
    in recurrent laryngeal nerve blocks,
        131, 131f
Cutaneous blocks, 90–105, 202–204
    in children, 202–204
    continuous
        femoral, 172–173
        psoas compartment (lumbar plexus),
            170–171
    fascia iliacus block, 93–95, 202
    femoral block, 96–99, 203–204
    posterior lumbar plexus (psoas) block,
        90–92
Cutaneous nerve
    of calf, 103f
    in 3-in-1 block, 98f
    lateral femoral, 64f
    in musculocutaneous nerve blocks, 26t
    in sciatic nerve blocks, 72, 75f
Cutaneous nerve blocks
    for arteriovenous fistula
        of forearm, 26t
Cutaneous radial nerve
    in truncular blocks, 23

**D**

Dalens' technique
    in axillary block, 194
Debridement, 67
Digital blocks, 23–24
Digital sheath blocks
    terminal blocks, 59–61
Digits
    terminal blocks of, 23, 59–61
Distal blocks, 18
Dorsal nerve, 23–24
Droperidol
    in airway blocks, 126
    in peripheral nerve blocks, 5
Dupuytren disease
    axillary blocks for, 26t

**E**

Elbow blocks
    olecranon process in, 49, 49f
Elbows
    radial nerve blocks in, 18
    surgery of
        axillary blocks for, 25, 40, 152
        subclavicular blocks for, 25
        truncular and terminal nerve blocks
            for, 23, 25, 46, 49–53
    ulnar neurolysis at
        axillary blocks for, 26t
Elderly
    midazolam for
        in peripheral nerve blocks, 5
    retrobulbar hemorrhage risk in
        during peribulbar block, 114
EMLA cream, 4
    in pediatric peripheral blocks, 184
    side effects of, 181
Epicondylitis
    axillary blocks for, 26t
Epidural spread
    in continuous psoas compartment
        (lumbar plexus) blocks, 171
Epinephrine, 13
    in airway blocks, 126
    in fascia iliacus blocks, 94, 95
    in ilioinguinal blocks, 214
    in intercostal blocks, 118
    in lower extremity blocks, 69
    in pediatric peripheral blocks, 181, 187
    in penile blocks, 211
    in sciatic nerve blocks, 88
    side effects of, 13, 181
    in superior laryngeal nerve blocks, 129
    in thoracic paravertebral blocks, 135
Eyes
    surgery of
        peribulbar blocks for, 112

**F**

Facial nerve paralysis
    after cervical blocks, 110

Fascia iliacus blocks, 93–95, 202
    anatomic landmarks, 93, 93f, 202
    approach and technique, 94, 94f, 202
    in children, 202
    contrast medium spray in, 93, 93f
    indications for, 93, 202
    needles, 93, 94, 202
    patient position, 93, 202
    sedation for, 94
    systemic toxicity of, 95
Feet
    surgery of
        ankle blocks for, 68, 206
        sciatic nerve blocks for, 68, 198, 199
Femoral blocks, 96–99
    anatomic landmarks, 96, 96f, 203, 203f
    approach and technique, 97, 97f, 204,
        204f
    continuous, 172–173, 172f
    indications for, 96, 203
    needles, 96, 203
    patient position, 96, 203
    pediatric particularities, 204
    saphenous nerve in, 96f
    volume, 96, 203
Femoral cutaneous nerve, 65–66
Femoral fractures
    femoral block for, 203
Femoral nerves, 64f, 65–66
    in femoral blocks, 96, 96f, 97, 98, 98f
    and fascia iliacus block, 93
    in foot, 103f
    in 3-in-1 block, 98f
    in sciatic nerve blocks, 79f, 80f
Femur
    fractures of
        3-in-1 block for, 66t
        lumbar plexus block for, 66t
Fentanyl
    in airway blocks, 126
    in peripheral nerve blocks, 5
Fingers
    motor response of
        in continuous wrist blocks, 156
    surgery of
        continuous axillary blocks for, 152
        continuous wrist blocks for, 156
Flumazenil, 5
Foot
    calcaneal nerve in, 103f
    cutaneous innervation of, 103f
    femoral nerve in, 103f
    lateral plantar nerve in, 103f
    medial plantar nerve in, 103f
    motor innervation of, 65
    peroneal nerve in, 103f
    plantar nerve in, 103f
    saphenous nerve in, 66, 103f
    sensory innervation of, 65, 66
    superficial peroneal nerve in, 65
    sural nerve in, 65

Needles (*contd.*)
for interscalene blocks, 30
nerve stimulators, 9
for parascalene blocks, 190
for pediatric peripheral blocks, 186
for peribulbar blocks, 112, 114
for posterior lumbar plexus (psoas)
    blocks, 90, 91
for recurrent laryngeal nerve blocks,
    131
for sciatic nerve blocks
    anterior approach, 79, 82
    lateral approach, 87, 198
    parasacral approach, 72
    posterior approach, 75, 85, 196, 196f
Stimuplex. See Stimuplex needles
for superior laryngeal nerve blocks, 129
for supraclavicular blocks, 36
for thoracic paravertebral blocks, 134
for truncular blocks, 46, 49, 54, 59
Nerve compression
in ankle blocks, 207
Nerve sheath blocks
continuous, 176
Nerve stimulators, 8–10
in ankle blocks, 207
in axillary blocks, 22, 22f, 40, 41, 41f,
    192
in continuous infraclavicular blocks, 149
in continuous interscalene blocks, 144,
    144f
in continuous sciatic blocks, 168
in femoral blocks, 97, 97f
in high humeral blocks, 10
in lower extremity blocks, 64
needles for, 9
in pediatric peripheral blocks, 186
peripheral, 8, 8f
    in sciatic nerve blocks, 72
in posterior lumbar plexus (psoas)
    blocks, 90–91
in sciatic nerve blocks, 10, 76, 76f, 82,
    87
in supraclavicular blocks, 37
in truncular blocks, 47–48, 58
in ulnar blocks, 51–52, 51f 52f
vs. paresthesia, 8–9, 10
in wrist blocks, 56, 56f

## O
Obesity
in cervical blocks, 110
in posterior lumbar plexus blocks, 92
in sciatic nerve blocks, 82
in supraclavicular blocks, 37
Obturator nerves, 64f, 65, 66
in fascia iliacus blocks, 93
in femoral blocks, 98, 98f
in hip, 66
in 3-in-1 blocks, 98f
in sciatic nerve blocks, 74

Ocular perforation
in peribulbar block, 114
Olecranon process
in elbow blocks, 49, 49f
Opioids, 14
side effects of, 14

## P
Pain
from abdominal incisions
    intercostal block for, 118
from cholecystectomy
    thoracic paravertebral block for, 134
continuous psoas compartment (lumbar
    plexus) block for, 170
from fractured ribs
    intercostal block for, 118
intraoperative
    parascalene block for, 190
postoperative. See Postoperative pain
from thoracotomy
    thoracic paravertebral block for, 134
from thoracotomy incisions
    intercostal block for, 118
Palmer cutaneous nerve, 23–24, 24f
Paraphimosis
penile block for, 211
Parascalene block
in children, 190–191
    anatomic landmarks, 190, 190f
    approach and technique, 191, 191f
    contraindications for, 190
    indications for, 190
    patient position, 190
    pediatric peculiarities of, 191
    side effects of, 190
Paresis
after peribulbar blocks, 114
Patient-controlled analgesia
in continuous interscalene blocks, 144
Patient instructions
for continuous sciatic blocks
    posterior popliteal approach, 165
for hand and wrist surgery, 27
for interscalene blocks, 31
for pediatric peripheral blocks, 184
for peripheral nerve blocks, 5
Pediatric cutaneous blocks, 202–204
Pediatric peripheral blocks, 180–214
anatomy of, 184
ankle, 206–207
axillary, 194
complications of
    adjuvant-related, 181
cutaneous, 202–204
    fascia iliaca compartment, 202
    femoral, 203–204
equipment for, 186, 187
ilioinguinal, 214
indications for, 180–181
local anesthesia for, 186–187, 186t

parascalene, 190–191
penile, 210–211
pharmacology of, 184
psychology of, 184
recommendations for, 186
risk/benefit ratio, 181
sciatic nerve, 196–199
    lateral approach, 198
    popliteal approach, 199
    posterior approach, 196–197
sedation for, 187
toxicity of, 180–181
Pelvic sphlanic nerve
in sciatic nerve blocks, 72
Penile block
in children, 210–211
    anatomic landmarks, 210
    approach and technique, 210, 210f
    indications for, 210
    patient position, 210
    pediatric particularities, 211
Peribulbar blocks, 112–115
anatomic landmarks, 112
approach and technique, 112–114, 112f
    113f
        inferotemporal pericone injection,
            112, 112f
        medial canthus (caruncula) approach,
            115
        superonasal pericone injection, 113,
            113f
complications of, 114–115
evaluation of, 114
indications for, 112
local anesthesia for, 112
patient position, 112
sedation for, 114
Peripheral nerve blocks
benefits of, 4t
contraindications for, 4
evaluation of, 5
indications for, 4
informed consent for, 4
patient instruction for, 5
patient monitoring for, 4
postoperative follow-up for, 5
risks of, 4t
sedation in, 5
steps for, 4–5
Peripheral nerve stimulators, 8, 8f
in sciatic nerve blocks, 72
Peroneal nerve, 64f, 65
in ankle blocks, 102, 102f, 103–104,
    104, 105
in foot, 103f
in sciatic nerve blocks, 72, 73f, 76f, 81f
Phenylephrine
in airway blocks, 126
Phimosis
penile blocks for, 211
Phrenic nerve, 20

Phrenic nerve paralysis
  after cervical blocks, 110
  after continuous interscalene blocks,
    145
Physical therapy
  postoperative
    continuous infraclavicular block for,
      148
    continuous interscalene block for, 144
Plantar nerve, 64f
  in foot, 103f
Plexus
  irritation of
    in continuous interscalene blocks, 145
Pneumothorax
  after continuous interscalene blocks, 145
  after intercostal blocks, 121
  after subclavicular blocks, 25
  after supraclavicular blocks, 37
Posterior femoral cutaneous nerve, 64f, 75f
  in sciatic nerve blocks, 72
Posterior interosseous nerve
  in truncular blocks, 26t
Posterior lumbar plexus (psoas) blocks,
    90–92
  anatomic landmarks, 90, 90f
  approach and technique, 91, 91f
  indications for, 90
  needles, 90, 91
  patient position, 90
Posterior tibial nerve
  in ankle blocks, 102, 102f
  block of, 103
Postoperative analgesia. See Postoperative
    pain
Postoperative anticoagulation
  continuous psoas compartment (lumbar
    plexus) block alternative to
  for postoperative anticoagulation
Postoperative pain
  axillary blocks for, 194
  continuous axillary blocks for, 152
  continuous femoral blocks for, 172
  continuous infraclavicular blocks for,
    148
  continuous nerve sheath blocks for, 176
  continuous psoas compartment (lumbar
    plexus) blocks for, 170
  continuous sciatic blocks for
    lateral popliteal approach, 166, 168
    parasacral approach, 162
    posterior popliteal approach, 164
  continuous wrist blocks for, 156
  fascia iliacus blocks for, 93, 94, 95
  lumbar plexus block for, 66t
  parascalene blocks for, 190
  pediatric peripheral blocks for, 180–181
  penile blocks for, 211
Postoperative physical therapy
  continuous infraclavicular blocks for,
    148

continuous interscalene blocks for, 144
continuous wrist blocks for, 156
Psoas block
  posterior. See Posterior lumbar plexus
    (psoas) block
Psoas compartment, 91, 91f
Psoas compartment (lumbar plexus) block
  continuous, 170–171, 170f
Pudendal nerve
  in sciatic nerve blocks, 72, 74

**Q**
Quadriceps muscle
  biopsy of
    3-in-1 block for, 66t

**R**
Radial nerve, 21, 23
  anastamoses, 18t
  in axillary blocks, 42f
  in brachial plexus blocks, 19f
  in continuous wrist blocks, 156, 159,
    159f, 160
  cutaneous
    in truncular blocks, 23
  in interscalene blocks, 31
  in truncular blocks, 26t, 48, 48f
    at elbow, 50, 50f
    high humeral approach, 47
    at wrist, 53, 53f, 58, 58f
Radial nerve blocks
  axilla
    forearm sensory block, 18
  in elbow, 18
  for trigger finger, 26t
Raj's anterior approach
  of sciatic nerve, 65, 82, 83f
Recurrent laryngeal nerve blocks
  anatomic landmarks, 131
  approach and technique, 131, 133f
  contraindications for, 132
  cricothyroid membrane in, 131, 131f
  indications for, 131
  patient position, 131
Respiratory insufficiency
  and interscalene block, 31
  and parascalene block, 190
Retrobulbar block, 114
Retrobulbar hemorrhage
  in peribulbar block, 114
Ribs
  fractured
    intercostal block for, 118
Ropivacaine
  in continuous peripheral blocks, 140,
    141
  in continuous wrist blocks, 156
  in fascia iliacus blocks, 94
  in lower extremity blocks, 69
  in peribulbar blocks, 115
  toxicity of, 12

**S**
Sacral plexus, 72
  in continuous sciatic blocks
    parasacral approach, 162
Saphenous nerve, 64f, 66
  in ankle blocks, 102, 102f, 104, 207
  block of, 103–104
  in femoral blocks, 96f
  in foot, 103f
  in 3-in-1 block, 98f
Saphenous vein stripping, 66t
Sciatic nerve, 64f, 75f, 79f, 80f, 94, 94f
  Beck's anterior approach, 65, 82, 83f
  Chelly's anterior approach, 65, 79f, 82,
    83f
Sciatic nerve blocks, 72–88, 196–199
  in ankles, 66t
  anterior approach, 79–83
  in children
    anatomic landmarks, 196, 199
    approach and technique, 196, 196f
    indications for, 196
    needles for, 196, 198, 199
    popliteal approach, 199
    posterior approach, 196–197
  common peroneal nerve in, 72, 73f
  continuous. See Continuous sciatic
    blocks
  contraindications for, 67
  cutaneous nerve in, 72, 75f
  femoral nerve in, 79f, 80f
  gluteal nerve in, 72
  lateral approach, 198
  lateral popliteal approach, 87–88
  in lower extremities, 68–69
  nerve stimulators, 10
  obturator nerve in, 74
  parasacral approach
    anatomic landmarks, 72
    approach and technique, 72, 73f
    indications for, 72
  pelvic sphlanic nerve in, 72
  peroneal nerve in, 72, 73f, 76f, 81f
  popliteal approach, 199
  posterior approach
    anatomic landmarks, 72, 73f
    approach and technique, 76, 76f
    indications for, 75
  posterior femoral cutaneous nerve in, 72
  posterior popliteal approach, 85–86
  pudendal nerve in, 72, 74
  superior gluteal nerve in, 72
  tibial nerve in, 72, 73f, 76f, 80f
Sciatic nerves
  characteristics of, 197
Sciatic plexus nerves, 65
Scleral buckle
  peribulbar block for, 112
Sedation
  for airway blocks, 126
  for cervical blocks, 110

continuous axillary block for, 152
continuous infraclavicular block for, 148
parascalene block for, 190
Upper extremity blocks
anatomic considerations, 18–19
brachial plexus nerve anastomosis, 18, 18t
global innervation, 18–19, 19f
nerve branching levels, 18
extension of, 19–24
indications for, 18–27, 26t
onset time, 12
surgical indications for, 25–27

Vagal nerve paralysis
after cervical blocks, 110
Vagus nerve
in airway blocks, 126
Vasoconstrictors
in pediatric peripheral blocks, 187
Ventricular fibrillation
after pediatric peripheral blocks, 180
Vitreoretinal surgery
peribulbar block for, 112
Vocal cord movement
evaluation of
recurrent laryngeal nerve block in, 131
superior laryngeal nerve block in, 130

Webril padding band, 122, 122f
Wrist
surgery of
axillary blocks for, 26
continuous wrist block for, 156
humeral blocks for, 26
synovial cyst of
axillary blocks for, 26t
truncular blocks for, 26t
Wrist blocks
continuous, 156–160
finger motor response, 156
truncular, 23, 54–58
ulnar nerve in, 56, 56f